50% OFF

Online CPC Prep Course!

By Mometrix

Dear Customer,

We consider it an honor and a privilege that you chose our CPC Study Guide. As a way of showing our appreciation and to help us better serve you, we are offering **50% off our online CPC Prep Course**. Many CPC courses are needlessly expensive and don't deliver enough value. With our course, you get access to the best CPC prep material, and **you only pay half price**.

We have structured our online course to perfectly complement your printed study guide. The CPC Prep Course contains **in-depth lessons** that cover all the most important topics, **400 practice questions** to ensure you feel prepared, and more than **250 digital flashcards**, so you can study while you're on the go.

Online CPC Prep Course

Topics Included:

- Current Procedural Terminology (CPT) Surgical Procedures
- Evaluation and Management (E/M)
- Anesthesia
- International Classifications of Diseases, 10th Revision, Clinical Modification (ICD-10-CM)
- Radiology
- Laboratory and Pathology
- Medicine
- Healthcare Common Procedure Coding System (HCPCS) Level II
- Coding Guidelines
- Compliance and Regulatory

Course Features:

- CPC Study Guide
  - Get content that complements our best-selling study guide.
- Full-Length Practice Tests
  - With 400 practice questions, you can test yourself again and again.
- Mobile Friendly
  - If you need to study on the go, the course is easily accessible from your mobile device.
- CPC Flashcards
  - Our course includes a flashcard mode with over 250 content cards to help you study.

To receive this discount, visit us at mometrix.com/university/cpc or simply scan this QR code with your smartphone. At the checkout page, enter the discount code: **cpc50off**

If you have any questions or concerns, please contact us at support@mometrix.com.

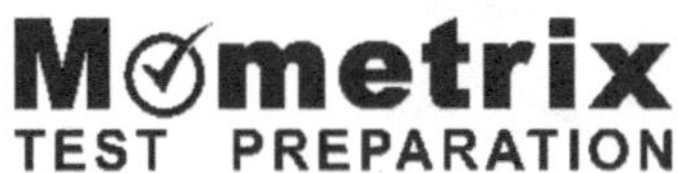

FREE Study Skills Videos/DVD Offer

Dear Customer,

Thank you for your purchase from Mometrix! We consider it an honor and a privilege that you have purchased our product and we want to ensure your satisfaction.

As part of our ongoing effort to meet the needs of test takers, we have developed a set of Study Skills Videos that we would like to give you for FREE. These videos cover our *best practices* for getting ready for your exam, from how to use our study materials to how to best prepare for the day of the test.

All that we ask is that you email us with feedback that would describe your experience so far with our product. Good, bad, or indifferent, we want to know what you think!

To get your FREE Study Skills Videos, you can use the **QR code** below, or send us an **email** at studyvideos@mometrix.com with *FREE VIDEOS* in the subject line and the following information in the body of the email:

- The name of the product you purchased.
- Your product rating on a scale of 1-5, with 5 being the highest rating.
- Your feedback. It can be long, short, or anything in between. We just want to know your impressions and experience so far with our product. (Good feedback might include how our study material met your needs and ways we might be able to make it even better. You could highlight features that you found helpful or features that you think we should add.)

If you have any questions or concerns, please don't hesitate to contact me directly.

Thanks again!

Sincerely,

Jay Willis
Vice President
jay.willis@mometrix.com
1-800-673-8175

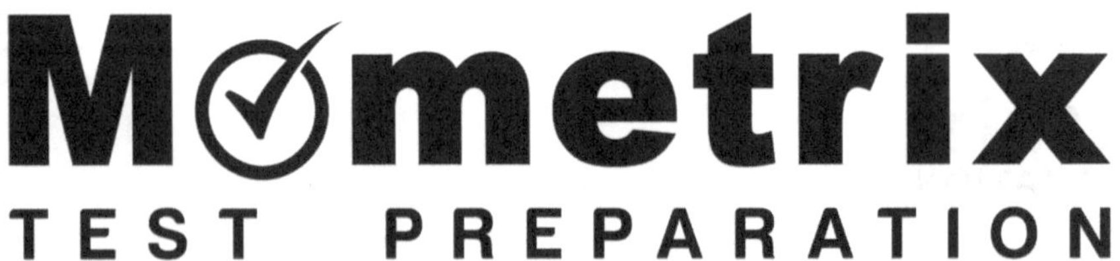

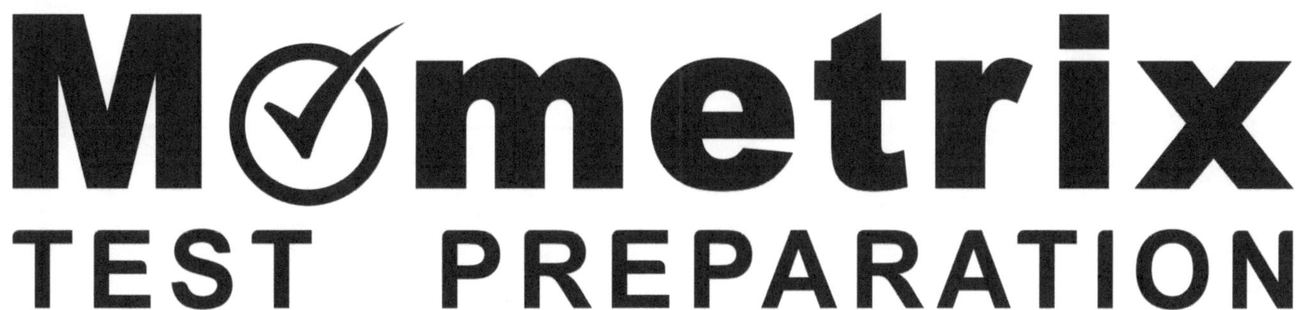

CPC

Study Guide 2024-2025

4 Full-Length Practice Tests

Secrets Exam Preparation for the AAPC Professional Coder Certification

5th Edition

CPC Study Guide - Full-Length Practice Tests, Secrets Exam Preparation for the AAPC Professional Coder Certification: [5th Edition]

Written and edited by Matthew Bowling

Printed in the United States of America

This paper meets the requirements of ANSI/NISO Z39.48-1992 (Permanence of Paper).

Paperback
ISBN 13: 978-1-5167-2697-4
ISBN 10: 1-5167-2697-9

Dear Future Exam Success Story

First of all, **THANK YOU** for purchasing Mometrix study materials!

Second, congratulations! You are one of the few determined test-takers who are committed to doing whatever it takes to excel on your exam. **You have come to the right place.** We developed these study materials with one goal in mind: to deliver you the information you need in a format that's concise and easy to use.

In addition to optimizing your guide for the content of the test, we've outlined our recommended steps for breaking down the preparation process into small, attainable goals so you can make sure you stay on track.

We've also analyzed the entire test-taking process, identifying the most common pitfalls and showing how you can overcome them and be ready for any curveball the test throws you.

Standardized testing is one of the biggest obstacles on your road to success, which only increases the importance of doing well in the high-pressure, high-stakes environment of test day. Your results on this test could have a significant impact on your future, and this guide provides the information and practical advice to help you achieve your full potential on test day.

Your success is our success

We would love to hear from you! If you would like to share the story of your exam success or if you have any questions or comments in regard to our products, please contact us at **800-673-8175** or **support@mometrix.com**.

Thanks again for your business and we wish you continued success!

Sincerely,
The Mometrix Test Preparation Team

Need more help? Check out our flashcards at:
http://mometrixflashcards.com/CPC

TABLE OF CONTENTS

Introduction

Thank you for purchasing this resource! You have made the choice to prepare yourself for a test that could have a huge impact on your future, and this guide is designed to help you be fully ready for test day. Obviously, it's important to have a solid understanding of the test material, but you also need to be prepared for the unique environment and stressors of the test, so that you can perform to the best of your abilities.

For this purpose, the first section that appears in this guide is the **Secret Keys**. We've devoted countless hours to meticulously researching what works and what doesn't, and we've boiled down our findings to the five most impactful steps you can take to improve your performance on the test. We start at the beginning with study planning and move through the preparation process, all the way to the testing strategies that will help you get the most out of what you know when you're finally sitting in front of the test.

We recommend that you start preparing for your test as far in advance as possible. However, if you've bought this guide as a last-minute study resource and only have a few days before your test, we recommend that you skip over the first two Secret Keys since they address a long-term study plan.

If you struggle with **test anxiety**, we strongly encourage you to check out our recommendations for how you can overcome it. Test anxiety is a formidable foe, but it can be beaten, and we want to make sure you have the tools you need to defeat it.

Secret Key #1 – Plan Big, Study Small

There's a lot riding on your performance. If you want to ace this test, you're going to need to keep your skills sharp and the material fresh in your mind. You need a plan that lets you review everything you need to know while still fitting in your schedule. We'll break this strategy down into three categories.

Information Organization

Start with the information you already have: the official test outline. From this, you can make a complete list of all the concepts you need to cover before the test. Organize these concepts into groups that can be studied together, and create a list of any related vocabulary you need to learn so you can brush up on any difficult terms. You'll want to keep this vocabulary list handy once you actually start studying since you may need to add to it along the way.

Time Management

Once you have your set of study concepts, decide how to spread them out over the time you have left before the test. Break your study plan into small, clear goals so you have a manageable task for each day and know exactly what you're doing. Then just focus on one small step at a time. When you manage your time this way, you don't need to spend hours at a time studying. Studying a small block of content for a short period each day helps you retain information better and avoid stressing over how much you have left to do. You can relax knowing that you have a plan to cover everything in time. In order for this strategy to be effective though, you have to start studying early and stick to your schedule. Avoid the exhaustion and futility that comes from last-minute cramming!

Study Environment

The environment you study in has a big impact on your learning. Studying in a coffee shop, while probably more enjoyable, is not likely to be as fruitful as studying in a quiet room. It's important to keep distractions to a minimum. You're only planning to study for a short block of time, so make the most of it. Don't pause to check your phone or get up to find a snack. It's also important to **avoid multitasking**. Research has consistently shown that multitasking will make your studying dramatically less effective. Your study area should also be comfortable and well-lit so you don't have the distraction of straining your eyes or sitting on an uncomfortable chair.

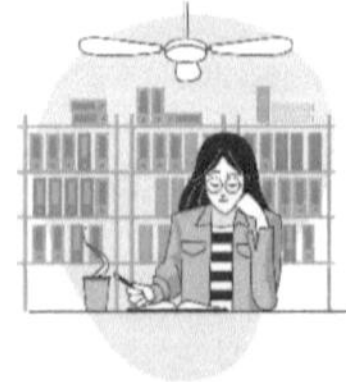

The time of day you study is also important. You want to be rested and alert. Don't wait until just before bedtime. Study when you'll be most likely to comprehend and remember. Even better, if you know what time of day your test will be, set that time aside for study. That way your brain will be used to working on that subject at that specific time and you'll have a better chance of recalling information.

Finally, it can be helpful to team up with others who are studying for the same test. Your actual studying should be done in as isolated an environment as possible, but the work of organizing the information and setting up the study plan can be divided up. In between study sessions, you can discuss with your teammates the concepts that you're all studying and quiz each other on the details. Just be sure that your teammates are as serious about the test as you are. If you find that your study time is being replaced with social time, you might need to find a new team.

Secret Key #2 – Make Your Studying Count

You're devoting a lot of time and effort to preparing for this test, so you want to be absolutely certain it will pay off. This means doing more than just reading the content and hoping you can remember it on test day. It's important to make every minute of study count. There are two main areas you can focus on to make your studying count.

Retention

It doesn't matter how much time you study if you can't remember the material. You need to make sure you are retaining the concepts. To check your retention of the information you're learning, try recalling it at later times with minimal prompting. Try carrying around flashcards and glance at one or two from time to time or ask a friend who's also studying for the test to quiz you.

To enhance your retention, look for ways to put the information into practice so that you can apply it rather than simply recalling it. If you're using the information in practical ways, it will be much easier to remember. Similarly, it helps to solidify a concept in your mind if you're not only reading it to yourself but also explaining it to someone else. Ask a friend to let you teach them about a concept you're a little shaky on (or speak aloud to an imaginary audience if necessary). As you try to summarize, define, give examples, and answer your friend's questions, you'll understand the concepts better and they will stay with you longer. Finally, step back for a big picture view and ask yourself how each piece of information fits with the whole subject. When you link the different concepts together and see them working together as a whole, it's easier to remember the individual components.

Finally, practice showing your work on any multi-step problems, even if you're just studying. Writing out each step you take to solve a problem will help solidify the process in your mind, and you'll be more likely to remember it during the test.

Modality

Modality simply refers to the means or method by which you study. Choosing a study modality that fits your own individual learning style is crucial. No two people learn best in exactly the same way, so it's important to know your strengths and use them to your advantage.

For example, if you learn best by visualization, focus on visualizing a concept in your mind and draw an image or a diagram. Try color-coding your notes, illustrating them, or creating symbols that will trigger your mind to recall a learned concept. If you learn best by hearing or discussing information, find a study partner who learns the same way or read aloud to yourself. Think about how to put the information in your own words. Imagine that you are giving a lecture on the topic and record yourself so you can listen to it later.

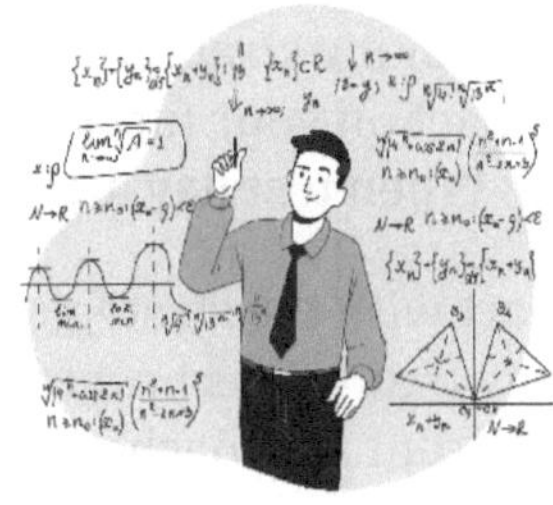

For any learning style, flashcards can be helpful. Organize the information so you can take advantage of spare moments to review. Underline key words or phrases. Use different colors for different categories. Mnemonic devices (such as creating a short list in which every item starts with the same letter) can also help with retention. Find what works best for you and use it to store the information in your mind most effectively and easily.

Secret Key #3 – Practice the Right Way

Your success on test day depends not only on how many hours you put into preparing, but also on whether you prepared the right way. It's good to check along the way to see if your studying is paying off. One of the most effective ways to do this is by taking practice tests to evaluate your progress. Practice tests are useful because they show exactly where you need to improve. Every time you take a practice test, pay special attention to these three groups of questions:

- The questions you got wrong
- The questions you had to guess on, even if you guessed right
- The questions you found difficult or slow to work through

This will show you exactly what your weak areas are, and where you need to devote more study time. Ask yourself why each of these questions gave you trouble. Was it because you didn't understand the material? Was it because you didn't remember the vocabulary? Do you need more repetitions on this type of question to build speed and confidence? Dig into those questions and figure out how you can strengthen your weak areas as you go back to review the material.

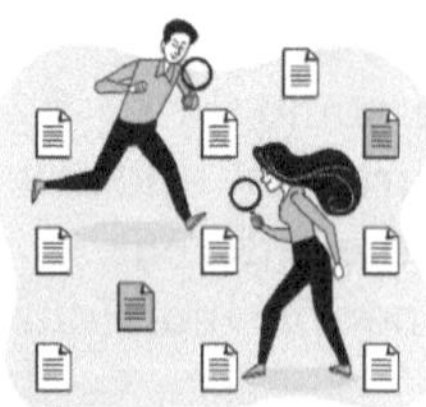

Additionally, many practice tests have a section explaining the answer choices. It can be tempting to read the explanation and think that you now have a good understanding of the concept. However, an explanation likely only covers part of the question's broader context. Even if the explanation makes perfect sense, **go back and investigate** every concept related to the question until you're positive you have a thorough understanding.

As you go along, keep in mind that the practice test is just that: practice. Memorizing these questions and answers will not be very helpful on the actual test because it is unlikely to have any of the same exact questions. If you only know the right answers to the sample questions, you won't be prepared for the real thing. **Study the concepts** until you understand them fully, and then you'll be able to answer any question that shows up on the test.

It's important to wait on the practice tests until you're ready. If you take a test on your first day of study, you may be overwhelmed by the amount of material covered and how much you need to learn. Work up to it gradually.

On test day, you'll need to be prepared for answering questions, managing your time, and using the test-taking strategies you've learned. It's a lot to balance, like a mental marathon that will have a big impact on your future. Like training for a marathon, you'll need to start slowly and work your way up. When test day arrives, you'll be ready.

Start with the strategies you've read in the first two Secret Keys—plan your course and study in the way that works best for you. If you have time, consider using multiple study resources to get different approaches to the same concepts. It can be helpful to see difficult concepts from more than one angle. Then find a good source for practice tests. Many times, the test website will suggest potential study resources or provide sample tests.

Practice Test Strategy

If you're able to find at least three practice tests, we recommend this strategy:

Untimed and Open-Book Practice

Take the first test with no time constraints and with your notes and study guide handy. Take your time and focus on applying the strategies you've learned.

Timed and Open-Book Practice

Take the second practice test open-book as well, but set a timer and practice pacing yourself to finish in time.

Timed and Closed-Book Practice

Take any other practice tests as if it were test day. Set a timer and put away your study materials. Sit at a table or desk in a quiet room, imagine yourself at the testing center, and answer questions as quickly and accurately as possible.

Keep repeating timed and closed-book tests on a regular basis until you run out of practice tests or it's time for the actual test. Your mind will be ready for the schedule and stress of test day, and you'll be able to focus on recalling the material you've learned.

Secret Key #4 – Pace Yourself

Once you're fully prepared for the material on the test, your biggest challenge on test day will be managing your time. Just knowing that the clock is ticking can make you panic even if you have plenty of time left. Work on pacing yourself so you can build confidence against the time constraints of the exam. Pacing is a difficult skill to master, especially in a high-pressure environment, so **practice is vital**.

Set time expectations for your pace based on how much time is available. For example, if a section has 60 questions and the time limit is 30 minutes, you know you have to average 30 seconds or less per question in order to answer them all. Although 30 seconds is the hard limit, set 25 seconds per question as your goal, so you reserve extra time to spend on harder questions. When you budget extra time for the harder questions, you no longer have any reason to stress when those questions take longer to answer.

Don't let this time expectation distract you from working through the test at a calm, steady pace, but keep it in mind so you don't spend too much time on any one question. Recognize that taking extra time on one question you don't understand may keep you from answering two that you do understand later in the test. If your time limit for a question is up and you're still not sure of the answer, mark it and move on, and come back to it later if the time and the test format allow. If the testing format doesn't allow you to return to earlier questions, just make an educated guess; then put it out of your mind and move on.

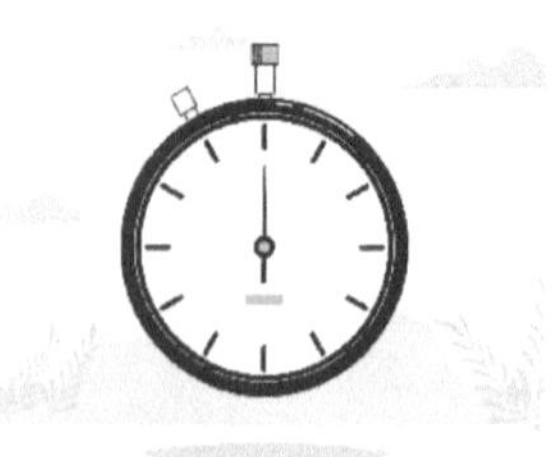

On the easier questions, be careful not to rush. It may seem wise to hurry through them so you have more time for the challenging ones, but it's not worth missing one if you know the concept and just didn't take the time to read the question fully. Work efficiently but make sure you understand the question and have looked at all of the answer choices, since more than one may seem right at first.

Even if you're paying attention to the time, you may find yourself a little behind at some point. You should speed up to get back on track, but do so wisely. Don't panic; just take a few seconds less on each question until you're caught up. Don't guess without thinking, but do look through the answer choices and eliminate any you know are wrong. If you can get down to two choices, it is often worthwhile to guess from those. Once you've chosen an answer, move on and don't dwell on any that you skipped or had to hurry through. If a question was taking too long, chances are it was one of the harder ones, so you weren't as likely to get it right anyway.

On the other hand, if you find yourself getting ahead of schedule, it may be beneficial to slow down a little. The more quickly you work, the more likely you are to make a careless mistake that will affect your score. You've budgeted time for each question, so don't be afraid to spend that time. Practice an efficient but careful pace to get the most out of the time you have.

Secret Key #5 – Have a Plan for Guessing

When you're taking the test, you may find yourself stuck on a question. Some of the answer choices seem better than others, but you don't see the one answer choice that is obviously correct. What do you do?

The scenario described above is very common, yet most test takers have not effectively prepared for it. Developing and practicing a plan for guessing may be one of the single most effective uses of your time as you get ready for the exam.

In developing your plan for guessing, there are three questions to address:

- When should you start the guessing process?
- How should you narrow down the choices?
- Which answer should you choose?

When to Start the Guessing Process

Unless your plan for guessing is to select C every time (which, despite its merits, is not what we recommend), you need to leave yourself enough time to apply your answer elimination strategies. Since you have a limited amount of time for each question, that means that if you're going to give yourself the best shot at guessing correctly, you have to decide quickly whether or not you will guess.

Of course, the best-case scenario is that you don't have to guess at all, so first, see if you can answer the question based on your knowledge of the subject and basic reasoning skills. Focus on the key words in the question and try to jog your memory of related topics. Give yourself a chance to bring the knowledge to mind, but once you realize that you don't have (or you can't access) the knowledge you need to answer the question, it's time to start the guessing process.

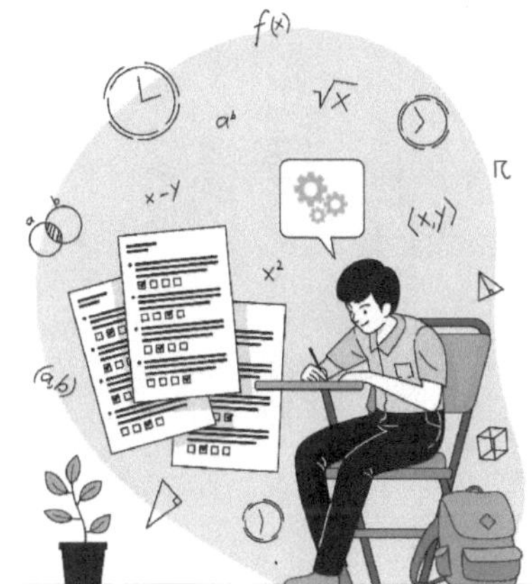

It's almost always better to start the guessing process too early than too late. It only takes a few seconds to remember something and answer the question from knowledge. Carefully eliminating wrong answer choices takes longer. Plus, going through the process of eliminating answer choices can actually help jog your memory.

Summary: Start the guessing process as soon as you decide that you can't answer the question based on your knowledge.

How to Narrow Down the Choices

The next chapter in this book (**Test-Taking Strategies**) includes a wide range of strategies for how to approach questions and how to look for answer choices to eliminate. You will definitely want to read those carefully, practice them, and figure out which ones work best for you. Here though, we're going to address a mindset rather than a particular strategy.

Your odds of guessing an answer correctly depend on how many options you are choosing from.

Number of options left	5	4	3	2	1
Odds of guessing correctly	20%	25%	33%	50%	100%

You can see from this chart just how valuable it is to be able to eliminate incorrect answers and make an educated guess, but there are two things that many test takers do that cause them to miss out on the benefits of guessing:

- Accidentally eliminating the correct answer
- Selecting an answer based on an impression

We'll look at the first one here, and the second one in the next section.

To avoid accidentally eliminating the correct answer, we recommend a thought exercise called **the $5 challenge**. In this challenge, you only eliminate an answer choice from contention if you are willing to bet $5 on it being wrong. Why $5? Five dollars is a small but not insignificant amount of money. It's an amount you could afford to lose but wouldn't want to throw away. And while losing $5 once might not hurt too much, doing it twenty times will set you back $100. In the same way, each small decision you make—eliminating a choice here, guessing on a question there—won't by itself impact your score very much, but when you put them all together, they can make a big difference. By holding each answer choice elimination decision to a higher standard, you can reduce the risk of accidentally eliminating the correct answer.

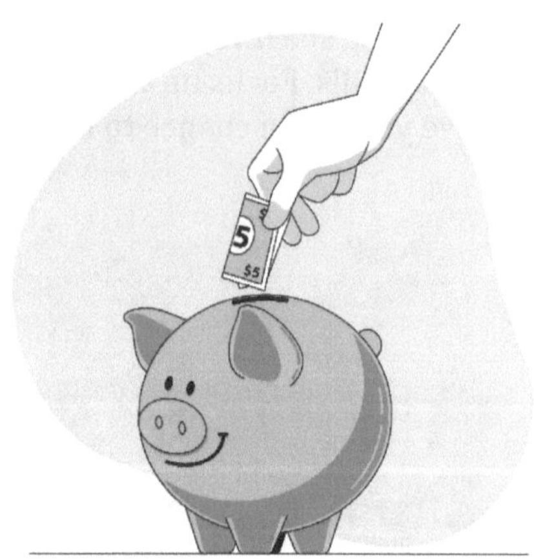

The $5 challenge can also be applied in a positive sense: If you are willing to bet $5 that an answer choice *is* correct, go ahead and mark it as correct.

Summary: Only eliminate an answer choice if you are willing to bet $5 that it is wrong.

Which Answer to Choose

You're taking the test. You've run into a hard question and decided you'll have to guess. You've eliminated all the answer choices you're willing to bet $5 on. Now you have to pick an answer. Why do we even need to talk about this? Why can't you just pick whichever one you feel like when the time comes?

The answer to these questions is that if you don't come into the test with a plan, you'll rely on your impression to select an answer choice, and if you do that, you risk falling into a trap. The test writers know that everyone who takes their test will be guessing on some of the questions, so they intentionally write wrong answer choices to seem plausible. You still have to pick an answer though, and if the wrong answer choices are designed to look right, how can you ever be sure that you're not falling for their trap? The best solution we've found to this dilemma is to take the decision out of your hands entirely. Here is the process we recommend:

Once you've eliminated any choices that you are confident (willing to bet $5) are wrong, select the first remaining choice as your answer.

Whether you choose to select the first remaining choice, the second, or the last, the important thing is that you use some preselected standard. Using this approach guarantees that you will not be enticed into selecting an answer choice that looks right, because you are not basing your decision on how the answer choices look.

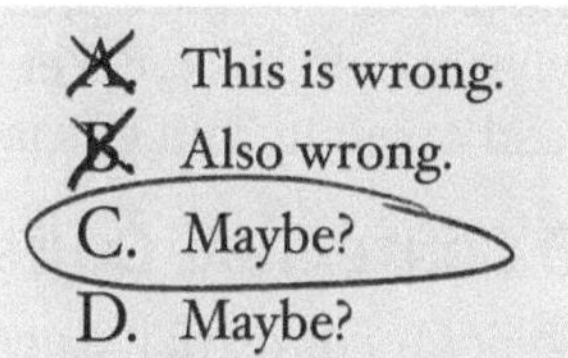

This is not meant to make you question your knowledge. Instead, it is to help you recognize the difference between your knowledge and your impressions. There's a huge difference between thinking an answer is right because of what you know, and thinking an answer is right because it looks or sounds like it should be right.

Summary: To ensure that your selection is appropriately random, make a predetermined selection from among all answer choices you have not eliminated.

Test-Taking Strategies

This section contains a list of test-taking strategies that you may find helpful as you work through the test. By taking what you know and applying logical thought, you can maximize your chances of answering any question correctly!

It is very important to realize that every question is different and every person is different: no single strategy will work on every question, and no single strategy will work for every person. That's why we've included all of them here, so you can try them out and determine which ones work best for different types of questions and which ones work best for you.

Question Strategies

✓ Read Carefully

Read the question and the answer choices carefully. Don't miss the question because you misread the terms. You have plenty of time to read each question thoroughly and make sure you understand what is being asked. Yet a happy medium must be attained, so don't waste too much time. You must read carefully and efficiently.

✓ Contextual Clues

Look for contextual clues. If the question includes a word you are not familiar with, look at the immediate context for some indication of what the word might mean. Contextual clues can often give you all the information you need to decipher the meaning of an unfamiliar word. Even if you can't determine the meaning, you may be able to narrow down the possibilities enough to make a solid guess at the answer to the question.

✓ Prefixes

If you're having trouble with a word in the question or answer choices, try dissecting it. Take advantage of every clue that the word might include. Prefixes can be a huge help. Usually, they allow you to determine a basic meaning. *Pre-* means before, *post-* means after, *pro-* is positive, *de-* is negative. From prefixes, you can get an idea of the general meaning of the word and try to put it into context.

✓ Hedge Words

Watch out for critical hedge words, such as *likely, may, can, sometimes, often, almost, mostly, usually, generally, rarely,* and *sometimes.* Question writers insert these hedge phrases to cover every possibility. Often an answer choice will be wrong simply because it leaves no room for exception. Be on guard for answer choices that have definitive words such as *exactly* and *always.*

✓ Switchback Words

Stay alert for *switchbacks.* These are the words and phrases frequently used to alert you to shifts in thought. The most common switchback words are *but, although,* and *however.* Others include *nevertheless, on the other hand, even though, while, in spite of, despite,* and *regardless of.* Switchback words are important to catch because they can change the direction of the question or an answer choice.

✅ FACE VALUE

When in doubt, use common sense. Accept the situation in the problem at face value. Don't read too much into it. These problems will not require you to make wild assumptions. If you have to go beyond creativity and warp time or space in order to have an answer choice fit the question, then you should move on and consider the other answer choices. These are normal problems rooted in reality. The applicable relationship or explanation may not be readily apparent, but it is there for you to figure out. Use your common sense to interpret anything that isn't clear.

Answer Choice Strategies

✅ ANSWER SELECTION

The most thorough way to pick an answer choice is to identify and eliminate wrong answers until only one is left, then confirm it is the correct answer. Sometimes an answer choice may immediately seem right, but be careful. The test writers will usually put more than one reasonable answer choice on each question, so take a second to read all of them and make sure that the other choices are not equally obvious. As long as you have time left, it is better to read every answer choice than to pick the first one that looks right without checking the others.

✅ ANSWER CHOICE FAMILIES

An answer choice family consists of two (in rare cases, three) answer choices that are very similar in construction and cannot all be true at the same time. If you see two answer choices that are direct opposites or parallels, one of them is usually the correct answer. For instance, if one answer choice says that quantity *x* increases and another either says that quantity *x* decreases (opposite) or says that quantity *y* increases (parallel), then those answer choices would fall into the same family. An answer choice that doesn't match the construction of the answer choice family is more likely to be incorrect. Most questions will not have answer choice families, but when they do appear, you should be prepared to recognize them.

✅ ELIMINATE ANSWERS

Eliminate answer choices as soon as you realize they are wrong, but make sure you consider all possibilities. If you are eliminating answer choices and realize that the last one you are left with is also wrong, don't panic. Start over and consider each choice again. There may be something you missed the first time that you will realize on the second pass.

✅ AVOID FACT TRAPS

Don't be distracted by an answer choice that is factually true but doesn't answer the question. You are looking for the choice that answers the question. Stay focused on what the question is asking for so you don't accidentally pick an answer that is true but incorrect. Always go back to the question and make sure the answer choice you've selected actually answers the question and is not merely a true statement.

✅ EXTREME STATEMENTS

In general, you should avoid answers that put forth extreme actions as standard practice or proclaim controversial ideas as established fact. An answer choice that states the "process should be used in certain situations, if..." is much more likely to be correct than one that states the "process should be discontinued completely." The first is a calm rational statement and doesn't even make a definitive, uncompromising stance, using a hedge word *if* to provide wiggle room, whereas the second choice is far more extreme.

⊘ Benchmark

As you read through the answer choices and you come across one that seems to answer the question well, mentally select that answer choice. This is not your final answer, but it's the one that will help you evaluate the other answer choices. The one that you selected is your benchmark or standard for judging each of the other answer choices. Every other answer choice must be compared to your benchmark. That choice is correct until proven otherwise by another answer choice beating it. If you find a better answer, then that one becomes your new benchmark. Once you've decided that no other choice answers the question as well as your benchmark, you have your final answer.

⊘ Predict the Answer

Before you even start looking at the answer choices, it is often best to try to predict the answer. When you come up with the answer on your own, it is easier to avoid distractions and traps because you will know exactly what to look for. The right answer choice is unlikely to be word-for-word what you came up with, but it should be a close match. Even if you are confident that you have the right answer, you should still take the time to read each option before moving on.

General Strategies

⊘ Tough Questions

If you are stumped on a problem or it appears too hard or too difficult, don't waste time. Move on! Remember though, if you can quickly check for obviously incorrect answer choices, your chances of guessing correctly are greatly improved. Before you completely give up, at least try to knock out a couple of possible answers. Eliminate what you can and then guess at the remaining answer choices before moving on.

⊘ Check Your Work

Since you will probably not know every term listed and the answer to every question, it is important that you get credit for the ones that you do know. Don't miss any questions through careless mistakes. If at all possible, try to take a second to look back over your answer selection and make sure you've selected the correct answer choice and haven't made a costly careless mistake (such as marking an answer choice that you didn't mean to mark). This quick double check should more than pay for itself in caught mistakes for the time it costs.

⊘ Pace Yourself

It's easy to be overwhelmed when you're looking at a page full of questions; your mind is confused and full of random thoughts, and the clock is ticking down faster than you would like. Calm down and maintain the pace that you have set for yourself. Especially as you get down to the last few minutes of the test, don't let the small numbers on the clock make you panic. As long as you are on track by monitoring your pace, you are guaranteed to have time for each question.

⊘ Don't Rush

It is very easy to make errors when you are in a hurry. Maintaining a fast pace in answering questions is pointless if it makes you miss questions that you would have gotten right otherwise. Test writers like to include distracting information and wrong answers that seem right. Taking a little extra time to avoid careless mistakes can make all the difference in your test score. Find a pace that allows you to be confident in the answers that you select.

⊘ Keep Moving

Panicking will not help you pass the test, so do your best to stay calm and keep moving. Taking deep breaths and going through the answer elimination steps you practiced can help to break through a stress barrier and keep your pace.

Final Notes

The combination of a solid foundation of content knowledge and the confidence that comes from practicing your plan for applying that knowledge is the key to maximizing your performance on test day. As your foundation of content knowledge is built up and strengthened, you'll find that the strategies included in this chapter become more and more effective in helping you quickly sift through the distractions and traps of the test to isolate the correct answer.

Now that you're preparing to move forward into the test content chapters of this book, be sure to keep your goal in mind. As you read, think about how you will be able to apply this information on the test. If you've already seen sample questions for the test and you have an idea of the question format and style, try to come up with questions of your own that you can answer based on what you're reading. This will give you valuable practice applying your knowledge in the same ways you can expect to on test day.

Good luck and good studying!

Current Procedural Terminology (CPT) Surgical Procedures

Transform passive reading into active learning! After immersing yourself in this chapter, put your comprehension to the test by taking a quiz. The insights you gained will stay with you longer this way. Scan the QR code to go directly to the chapter quiz interface for this study guide. If you're using a computer, simply visit the bonus page at **mometrix.com/bonus948/cpc** and click the Chapter Quizzes link.

General Procedures and the Integumentary System

Integumentary System

The integumentary system is made up primarily of the **skin,** including its multiple layers. Those layers include the **epidermis**, the outermost protective portion of the skin; the **dermis**, the middle layer, which consists of connective tissue, hair follicles, sweat glands, and nerve endings; and a layer of **subcutaneous tissue** that connects the outer layers to the muscle underneath and contains blood vessels and nerves. Hair and nails are also considered part of this system.

The integumentary system serves many key functions, including maintaining the body's homeostasis and shape, protecting internal tissues and organs from harm and infection, excreting waste via perspiration, and serving as a sensor for touch, pressure, heat, and cold.

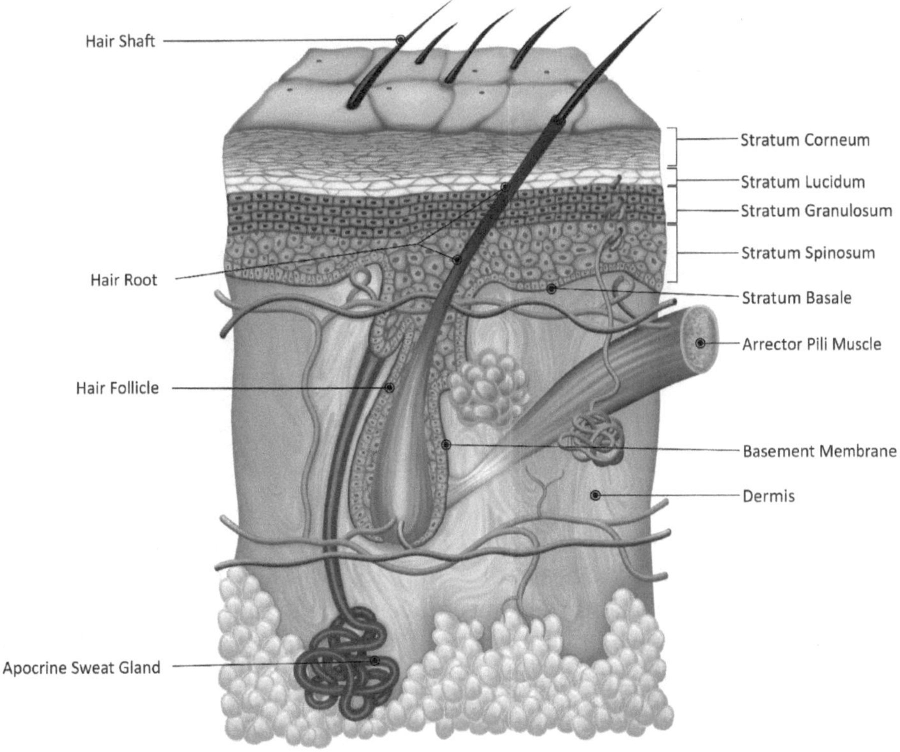

PROCEDURES

General surgical procedures and those involving the integumentary system are covered by CPT codes **10004** through **19499**, which are divided into related headings and subheadings throughout the section. Procedures relating to the skin and certain procedures of the breasts can be found here. In general, this includes:

- Performing biopsies of skin lesions
- Removing skin tags and other lesions
- Procedures involving fingernails and toenails
- Introducing substances into the skin
- Caring for and repairing wounds
- Skin grafts and skin replacement treatments
- Destruction of benign and malignant lesions
- Mohs micrographic surgery
- Mastectomies, breast repair, and breast reconstruction

Several codes, particularly those related to wound care and repair, are often included in surgical codes in later sections.

SKIN TAGS

Skin tags are small, soft, fleshy, and generally benign growths on the skin, often occurring on the eyelids, armpits, and neck, in the folds of the groin, underneath breasts, and in other places where the skin folds. Although skin tags are harmless, they can become irritated, and some consider them aesthetically unpleasing. Skin tags are typically removed with sharp tools (such as scissors or a scalpel), strangulation, electrocauterization, or chemical destruction.

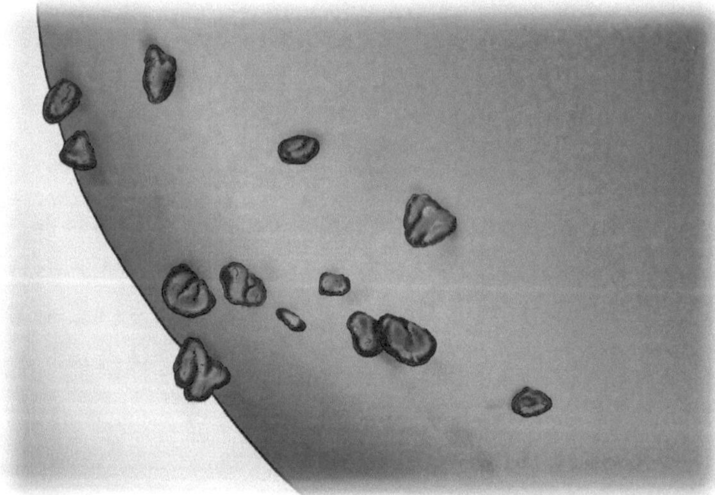

When coding for the removal of skin tags, use code **11200** for the first 15 tags removed, and then use the add-on code **11201** for each 10 tags after the first 15. Fractions of 10 still count toward the use of the add-on code. For example, if a physician removes 28 skin tags from a patient, the codes would be 11200 for the first 15, followed by two units of 11201: once for skin tags 16 through 25 and a second time for the remaining 3 skin tags. 15 + 10 + 3 = 28.

WOUND DEBRIDEMENT

Wound debridement is the medical removal of dead, damaged, infected, or otherwise nonviable tissue from an anatomical site. It is typically done to promote healing, prevent the spread of an infection, or remove debris or dead tissue from the area. Debridement can be done surgically, chemically, mechanically (such as with hydrotherapy), or by other methods.

When coding wound debridement, consider the surface area debrided, the depth of the wound that is being debrided, and the anatomical location of the wound being treated. If only a single wound is being debrided, use the code for the deepest level of tissue removed. If there are multiple wounds at differing depths, combine the surface areas of all wounds at the same depth separately from each other. For example, if a 6 cm^2 wound and a 12 cm^2 wound are debrided of subcutaneous tissue, while a separate 19 cm^2 wound is debrided to the bone, then only the 6 cm^2 and the 12 cm^2 wounds are added together, not all three.

SUBCUTANEOUS AND ACCESSORY STRUCTURES

FNA BIOPSY

A fine needle aspiration (FNA) biopsy, as defined by CPT, is a biopsy performed when material is aspirated with a fine needle and the cells are examined cytologically. The procedure involves using a thin needle to extract cells from abnormal tissue for analysis to aid in the diagnosis of a disease. This is typically performed on a lesion, cyst, or other type of mass located in or under the skin. An FNA biopsy can be done with or without imaging guidance.

FNA biopsies are covered by codes **10004** through **10012** and **10021**. When selecting the correct code, note what type of imaging guidance is used (if any), and how many lesions are biopsied. If multiple lesions are biopsied, **add-on codes** (indicated with a "**+**" next to the code number) will be needed in addition to the initial code. For example, two lesions biopsied while using ultrasound would be codes 10005 and 10006. If multiple types of imaging are used during the same session, report the additional codes with modifier 59. For example, one lesion with no guidance followed by one lesion with fluoroscopic guidance would be listed as 10007, 10021-59.

STANDARD TYPES OF BIOPSIES

CPT lists three types of biopsies, described as follows:

- **Tangential biopsies** are performed with a sharp blade, typically a scalpel, a **curette** (a sharp, hook-like scraping tool), or a flexible blade that cuts or shaves off a shallow sample of the tissue to be analyzed.
- **Punch biopsies** use a hollow cylindrical tool to remove a full-thickness sample of the skin and tissue, like taking a core sample from ice or wood. This procedure also includes closing the wound.
- **Incisional biopsies** are when the provider uses a sharp blade to remove a wedge or vertical incision to remove a full-thickness sample of tissue for diagnostic purposes. This procedure also includes closing the wound left behind.

When coding for biopsies, keep track of how many separate biopsies are performed. If different biopsies are all performed on the same lesion, use the primary codes for each different type. If different types of biopsies are performed on different lesions, report the CPT code of the biopsy with the highest relative value unit (RVU), followed by the add-on codes for each separate lesion. For example, if the method for obtaining tissue is a punch biopsy of a lesion, followed by an incisional biopsy on two other lesions, the reportable codes are 11106, +11107, and +11105.

Coding for Excision Procedures

Codes for excision procedures are distinguished by the lesion type (whether benign or cancerous), followed by the anatomical location of the lesion. For example, codes 11400 through 11406 are for a benign lesion on the trunk, legs, or arms.

Finally, when coding for excision, calculate the total diameter of the area being excised. This is done by adding together the lesion's size, plus the margins around it where it is excised. For example, if a 1 cm malignant lesion on a patient's arm is excised with margins of 1.5 cm on each side, add 1 cm + 1.5 cm + 1.5 cm = 4 cm, resulting in the code 11606.

Excision codes include simple closure of the wounds. If an intermediate or complex closure is required, it is coded separately.

Nails

Procedures in the CPT codebook that directly involve nails, nailbed, and the skin of the nail fold are covered by codes **11719** through **11765** and include the following:

- Trimming or debridement
- Removal of the actual hard surface of the nail, also known as **avulsion of the nail plate**
- Evacuation of **subungual hematomas,** or bruising or blood under a nail
- Excision of the nail and **nail matrix**, the area where the nail initially grows
- Biopsy of the entire nail
- Repair or reconstruction of the **nail bed,** the tissue underneath the actual hard surface of the nail, including tissue grafts
- Excisions to treat ingrown fingernails or toenails.

Pilonidal Cysts

A pilonidal cyst is a type of **cyst,** an abnormal sac filled with fluid or other material, that develops on a person's back, typically located at the base of the sacrum and just above the cleft of the buttocks. Pilonidal cysts typically contain pus, skin debris, and/or hair. They can become inflamed, infected, or painful without treatment. The CPT codes used for procedures to treat pilonidal cysts are **10080** through **10081** and **11770** through **11772**. The codes used depend on whether the cyst is **incised** (cut into) and drained or **excised** (removed) and the status of the cyst at the time of treatment.

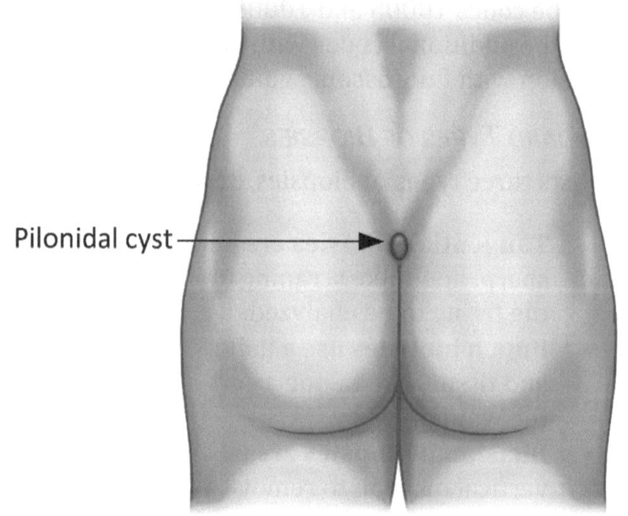

Wound Repairs

Types

Wound repair codes are used when a wound is closed via **sutures** (sewing the wound closed), staples, or tissue adhesives, either on their own or in concert. These codes do not apply if a wound is closed using only adhesive strips.

CPT classifies wound repairs into three different types:

- **Simple** repairs are used for superficial wounds, typically only including the epidermis, dermis, or subcutaneous tissue without additional involvement of deeper tissue. Simple repairs involve a single layer of closure, and they often include local anesthesia.
- **Intermediate** repairs include everything listed for simple repairs, but the wound requires layered closure of multiple layers of tissue or extensive cleaning or removal of foreign material. Intermediate repairs can include limited **undermining**, or when the wound extends in multiple directions under the opening but less than the maximum width of the wound's opening.
- **Complex** repairs involve wounds that, in addition to everything listed for intermediate repairs, include exposure of bone, cartilage, tendons, or other structures; debridement of wound edges due to trauma; extensive undermining (more than the maximum width of the wound's opening); involvement of the border between the skin and the rims of the ear, nostril, or lip; and/or the placement of retention sutures.

Coding

When selecting the correct wound repair code or codes, first determine the **location** of the wounds being repaired. Codes are grouped by anatomical location within the type of repair, such as simple or complex.

Next, check the **number** of wounds and what types they are. This is important for sequencing codes; the most complicated wound repair is considered to be the primary procedure, and any additional codes are secondary, requiring the use of the modifier 59.

Finally, check the **measurements** of the wounds that are being repaired. Procedures will give the wound sizes in centimeters. If multiple wounds are being repaired, add the total size of all wounds of the same type at the same anatomical location. For example, if a 3 cm and an 8 cm wound on the trunk are being closed with a simple repair, and a 6 cm wound on the trunk is being closed with a complex repair, add the two simple wounds together for a total of 11 cm.

Skin Graft Procedures

There are three key factors that must be considered when coding skin graft procedures, beginning with identifying the **source** of the graft. Most skin grafts are either **autografts**, which use tissue harvested or cultivated from the patient, or **skin substitutes**, which are from other people, animals, or synthetic skin substitutes. Next, consider the anatomical **location** of the graft. Like wound repair codes, skin graft codes cover a group of anatomical locations.

Finally, check the **size** of the graft. Grafts are coded with a primary code covering the first 100 cm^2 of a graft, with an add-on code for each additional 100 cm^2 or part thereof. So, for example, an epidermal autograft on the leg that covers 152 cm^2 would use codes 15110 and 15111: 15110 for the first 100 cm^2 and 15111 for the additional 52 cm^2.

This only applies to adults. When dealing with children or infants, code by percentage of body area covered by the graft.

Destruction

Destruction, in terms of medical procedures, is the ablation or elimination of various defects or lesions via a variety of methods. Methods include laser surgery, electrical cauterization, extreme cold, chemical removal, or surgical removal, and they include local anesthetic.

When coding destruction procedures, code for whether the procedure is targeting **benign** or **malignant** lesions, as well as the **number or size** of the lesion or lesions being removed. Some codes focus on the number of lesions removed (e.g., 17000 through 17004), whereas other codes are reported by obtaining the diameter in centimeters of a single lesion (e.g., 17260 through 17286).

MOHS MICROGRAPHIC SURGERY

Mohs micrographic surgery is a method used for removing complex or ill-defined skin cancer with histologic examination of the margins. The surgeon acts as both surgeon and pathologist, removing and analyzing the tissue in discrete pieces referred to as **blocks**, which is done in multiple progressively deeper layers called **stages.**

When a provider performs a Mohs surgery, keep track of the number of blocks and the number of stages. Codes **17311** and **17313** are used to code the first **stage**, including the first five blocks, with add-on codes 17312 and 17314 covering additional stages. The add-on code **17315** is used for additional blocks. Therefore, if a Mohs surgery is done on the trunk with four blocks in the first stage and seven blocks in the second, the codes used would be 17313 (first stage), 17314 (second stage with the first five blocks), and 17315 (the additional two blocks on the second stage).

BREASTS

CODES AND PROCEDURES

Procedures that involve the **breast**, here defined as tissues found within the human mammary glands in males and females, are covered by codes **19000** through 19499. The procedures covered by this section include the following:

- Aspiration of cysts located in the breast
- Biopsies of lesions or abnormal tissue found in the breast
- Excision of abnormal tissues from the breast, milk duct, or nipple
- Introduction of localization devices, primarily for cancer treatment
- Mastectomies
- Breast repair and reconstruction, including the insertion of implanted prosthetics.

Several of these procedures, particularly biopsies and introduction procedures, will include some form of imaging guidance (such as ultrasound or MRI) in the code.

MASTECTOMY PROCEDURES

CPT codes cover three different types of mastectomies, which are differentiated by the type and quantity of tissue removed during the procedure.

A **partial** mastectomy only removes a portion of the breast tissue from one or both breasts. This is typically the least extreme type of mastectomy.

A **simple, complete** mastectomy involves the complete removal of all breast tissue from the area and may include removal of the skin and/or nipple.

A **radical** mastectomy not only completely removes the breast tissue and nipple, but also removes the axillary lymph nodes, internal mammary lymph nodes, and/or pectoral muscle tissue. If only some lymph nodes are removed and the pectoral muscle tissue is left intact, a modified, radical mastectomy may be reported.

These are typically used for the treatment or prevention of breast cancer. If the removal is performed for a reduction or to treat gynecomastia, different codes will be used. In addition, codes used in this section are used for single breasts. If the procedure involves both breasts, append modifier 50 to the CPT code.

Musculoskeletal System

Musculoskeletal System

The musculoskeletal system is made up of two interlinked systems: the **muscular system,** which consists of the body's muscles, and the **skeletal system**, which consists of the body's bones. **Muscle** is soft tissue made up of protein filaments that can contract and relax when triggered by nerve impulses. Although there are three types of muscle in the human body, this section will focus on **skeletal muscles,** or muscles attached to the skeleton. **Bones,** meanwhile, are dense and hard tissue made up of specialized cells in a calcium matrix. The skeleton can be divided into two major regions: the **axial** skeleton, which includes the skull, spine, rib cage, and sternum; and the **appendicular** skeleton, which includes the limbs, hands, feet, hips, and shoulders. This section also includes procedures involving **joints,** or places where bones meet and are linked together via connective tissue.

Many of the musculoskeletal system's major functions focus on the body's movement, posture, and shape. The body's skeleton provides a sturdy framework for the rest of the body's systems, and protects vital organs from damage. Meanwhile, the body's muscles allow the body to move and balance, and they define its shape and retain body heat.

Procedures

Procedures involving the musculoskeletal system are covered by codes **20100** through **29999**, which are divided into related headings and subheadings throughout the section. Most of the headings are focused on a single anatomical location (e.g., head, hands, pelvis, hips), and they will often contain similar procedures.

Procedures in this section include the following:

- Incisions and drainage of abscesses
- Excision of tumors or tissue, including **fasciotomy** (the cutting of connective tissue)
- **Radical resection**, or extensive removal of a tumor with significant margins of normal tissue
- Introduction of drugs or substances into joints
- Repair and reconstruction procedures, including prosthetics
- Treatment of fractures and dislocations
- **Manipulation**, or manual, physical movement of the body for treatment
- **Arthrodesis**, or surgical immobilization of a bone or joint
- **Amputation**, or surgical removal of part or all of a limb or extremity
- Applications of casts and other immobilizing devices
- **Arthroscopic** procedures, in which a thin, flexible scope enters a joint space for surgery or investigation.

Open, Closed, and Percutaneous Treatment of Fractures

CPT uses specific terms when discussing procedures treating fractures. **Closed treatment** is when a fracture is treated without surgically opening the location. Typically, this involves either manipulation or traction of the site. **Open treatment** is when the fractured bone is either surgically exposed for visualization or treatment, or when an area near the fracture is opened to insert a fixation device across the site. **Percutaneous treatment**, or **percutaneous skeletal fixation**, is when the fracture is neither open nor closed. Instead, fixation devices (such as pins) are inserted through the skin, typically while using x-ray imaging guidance. This terminology has no bearing on the type of fracture, merely on the treatment type.

Traumatic Wounds

Traumatic wounds, meaning wounds resulting from penetrative trauma such as stabs and gunshots, often involve surgical exploration, enlargement, dissection, and/or debridement of the wound and its opening in order to remove foreign bodies, and repair minor subcutaneous and muscular blood vessels that do not require additional dedicated treatment. These types of procedures can be reported with CPT codes 20100 through 20103.

However, if repairs are done using a thoracotomy or laparotomy, then those codes are reported instead. In addition, if the wound or wounds do not require exploration or enlargement, report the wound repair codes used in the integumentary system instead.

Trigger Points

A trigger point is a persistent and often painful knot of muscle, typically located along the back, neck, shoulders, or spine, that does not relax along with the rest of the muscle. Trigger points often accompany certain conditions such as an injury; fibromyalgia; or chronic neck, jaw, or lower back pain. When a trigger point is treated, a muscle-relaxing agent such as lidocaine or a corticosteroid may be injected into the site. A physician may also opt to insert a dry needle into the site, causing the muscle to relax and release the knot.

When coding trigger point injections (CPT codes 20552 and 20553) and needle insertions without injections (CPT codes 20560 and 20561), it is important to note how many **muscles** are being treated, not the number of actual injections or needle insertions. For example, if 6 injections or needles are inserted on one muscle, and 4 injections or needles are inserted on another, then the code selection would be based on the two muscle sites, not the 10 injections or needles. Additional codes will be required if imaging guidance is used during the treatment.

External Fixation Devices

External fixation devices are used to correct and stabilize fractures or other bone defects. External fixation devices are attached to the bone through the skin via nails or pins, and they are bound to a metal frame that rests against or around the skin. Most such devices fall into three types:

- A **halo**, which attaches to the skull and is used typically for thin skull osteology
- A **uniplane external fixation system**, which is attached to a single bone or surface
- A **multiplane external fixation system**, which is attached to multiple bones or surfaces

The type of device used varies depending on the severity, type, and location of the defect or fracture, and the procedure is usually done with anesthesia.

IMMOBILIZING DEVICES

Various immobilizing devices are used when treating fractures and dislocations in order to prevent further damage and to promote healing. CPT covers three different types of immobilization devices:

- A **cast**, a protective shell made up of plastic, plaster, or fiberglass, designed to protect the damaged location
- A **splint**, a length of hard material placed along a limb and then secured with bandages
- **Strapping**, overlapping strips of adhesive tape or bandages wrapped around the area

When coding the use of immobilizing devices such as these, the initial cast used during part of a treatment is not coded. If it is performed afterward, or if it is separate from a treatment, then it should be coded. In addition, if the cast application or strapping is provided as the only initial care, then code **99070** should be used in addition to the relevant evaluation and management (E/M) code.

ENDOSCOPIC AND ARTHROSCOPIC PROCEDURES

Endoscopic procedures involve the use of a slender, flexible tube equipped with a light source, camera, and other tools (referred to as an **endoscope**) into a space inside the body. Endoscopic procedures are used for diagnostic or surgical purposes and are considered minimally invasive. Any surgical endoscopic procedure will, by necessity, include the services used in a diagnostic endoscopy; if there is a surgery involved, do not code a diagnostic endoscopy as well unless it is a completely separate service.

Arthroscopic procedures are a subset of endoscopies in which a scope is inserted into a joint for treatment and diagnosis. Arthroscopies can be performed on every major joint in the body, and they are listed in almost all sections of the musculoskeletal system. If an arthroscopy is performed with an **arthrotomy,** or surgical exploration, add modifier 51 to the arthroscopy code.

HEAD

Procedures involving the head (not including the skull) typically cover a few key anatomical sites. Common procedure sites on the head include the following:

- The **maxilla**, which forms the roof of the mouth and part of the eye sockets and nasal cavity
- The **mandibular rami,** the portion of the jawbone that curves upward behind the teeth
- The **temporomandibular joint**, the joint where the jawbone connects to the rest of the skull
- The **orbitals,** or the sections of bone that form the eye sockets
- The **scalp,** or the soft tissue on top of the head
- The **face,** which is typically involved in repair and reconstruction

CODING FOR EXCISION OF NECK AND THORAX

When coding excision procedures on the soft tissue of the neck and the thorax, there are several factors to take into account:

First, check the **location** of the procedure, whether it is in the neck or the **chest wall,** which is made up of the ribs and sternum. Excision codes for the neck and the chest wall have different factors that must be taken into account.

For neck excision codes, check the **size** of the tumor being removed, which should be listed in centimeters (cm). In addition, check the **depth** of the tumor, whether it is subcutaneous or **subfascial** (below the muscle).

For chest wall excision codes, check the **subject** of the removal, such as a tumor or an actual rib. In addition, check if a **lymphadenectomy**, or a dissection of the lymph nodes, is being performed in addition to the removal.

Coding of Excision of Back and Flank

Many of the codes dealing with the back and flank involve excision of soft tissue. Like most codes of similar procedures, there are a few key factors that must be accounted for in the procedure notes.

First, take the **depth** of the procedure into account, whether it is subcutaneous or subfascial. Afterward, check the **size** of the tumor being excised; CPT uses separate codes depending on if the mass is smaller than 5 cm or if it is 5 cm and larger.

When coding lesions that are cutaneous in origin (i.e., originating from the skin) and located on the back and flank, use codes located in the "Integumentary" section of CPT instead of codes in this section.

Spine

The **spinal column** comprises a stack of 33 bones, called **vertebrae**, that run from the skull to the tailbone. The spinal column is divided into four areas based on location. Starting from the skull, there are the **cervical vertebrae** (C1 through C7), which support the head and form the neck; the **thoracic vertebrae** (T1 through T12), which connect to the ribs and form the upper back; the **lumbar vertebrae** (L1 through L5), which form the lower back; and the **sacrum** (S1 through S5), which are fused together and connect to the pelvic bones to form the hips and the **coccyx**, or tailbone, which is actually another 4 bones fused together.

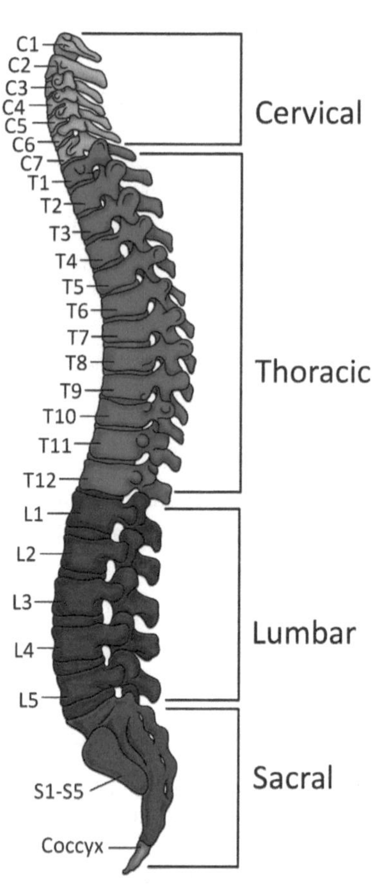

Each **vertebra** shares several key features. Starting from the anterior portion is the large **vertebral body**, a thick piece of bone that forms most of the spine's mass and supports the pads of connective tissue, which are known as **intervertebral discs.** Moving toward the posterior are the **pedicles**, which jut out from the body and link to the wing-like **transverse processes**. The transverse processes link into the **laminae,** which finally connect to the wedge-shaped **spinous processes**, which run along the posterior portion of the vertebrae. These arch-shaped protrusions help form the **spinal canal**, which the **spinal cord** runs through.

Spinal Arthrodesis Procedures

Spinal arthrodesis is the surgical fusion of two or more vertebrae, typically using grafted bone, in order to immobilize or stabilize vertebrae. Such procedures often include preparation procedures, a **discectomy** (the removal of the intervertebral disc), an **osteophytectomy** (the removal of any bone deposits or spurs), and possibly imaging guidance.

When coding these procedures, there are several key factors to take into account:

- First, confirm the **approach technique.** These procedures are divided up by how the spine is approached, such as through the back of the mouth or through the side of the neck.
- Next, confirm the **area of the spinal column** that is being immobilized. Depending on the approach, there may be a limited selection. An anterior transoral approach, for example, will only have the cervical vertebrae available to select from.
- After that, make note of the **number of interspaces** being immobilized. The **interspaces** are the spaces between vertebral bodies, so make sure not to confuse them with the vertebrae themselves. For example, the space between the C2 and C3 vertebrae is one interspace.

Spinal Instrumentation

Spinal instrumentation is the term used for prosthetic devices designed to support or stabilize damaged vertebrae and related structures. It may also include spinal fusion, which can span multiple vertebrae. Spinal instrumentation includes the following devices:

- **Non-segmental spinal instrumentation**, typically a rod that is connected at either end to the spine
- **Segmental spinal instrumentation**, similar to non-segmental spinal instrumentation but connected to additional bony attachments
- **Intervertebral biomechanical device**, a synthetic cage or mesh attached to the vertebral body
- **Arthroplasty,** a synthetic intervertebral disc

Be aware that many instrumentation insertions, reinsertions, and removal services may not be reported in conjunction with some CPT codes. On the other hand, some are only to be reported as a secondary code to another primary procedure performed. Therefore, pay close attention to the "Excludes" and "Includes" notes attached to each CPT code.

Coding for Excision of Abdomen

Most procedures involving the abdomen focus on excision of tumors and similar masses located in or on the **abdominal wall**, the band of muscular and connective tissue that encompasses the abdomen and the organs contained within. When coding these procedures, check the **depth**—subcutaneous or subfascial—because different depths require different codes. In addition, when coding these excision codes, check the **size** of the tumor being removed, which should be listed in centimeters (cm). Multiple tumors will require additional codes because each code is meant for a single tumor.

If the lesions have a **cutaneous origin**, meaning they originate in the skin and not the actual abdominal tissue, then you will need to use codes from the "Integumentary" section of CPT.

Coding Shoulder Procedures

The shoulder is a complex system of joints formed at the intersection of three bones: the humerus, the scapula, and the clavicle. Together, these three bones form the two joints of the shoulder: the **glenohumeral joint**, which is formed where the rounded head of the humerus slots into the concave portion of the scapula; and the **acromioclavicular joint**, which is where the highest point of the scapula meets the clavicle. The shoulder section also covers the various muscles and tendons that make up what is referred to as the **rotator cuff**, which holds the head of the humerus in place and allows the arm to be rotated above the head.

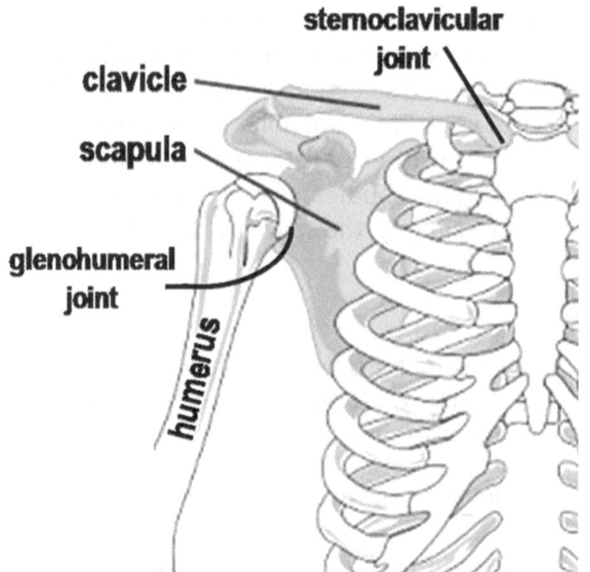

Coding Procedures of Arm and Elbow

The **humerus** is the long bone that forms the upper part of the arm, connecting the shoulder to the forearm. Codes relating to the humerus and elbow cover the **shaft** (the long central portion) and the **distal** (furthest from the center of the body) end of the humerus. The humerus, alongside the proximal ends of the **radius** (the thinner forearm bone) and the **ulna** (the thicker, longer forearm bone) form the **elbow joint.** This section also covers procedures involving the **olecranon process**, which is the thick, proximal head of the ulna that forms the "bump" on the elbow; as well as the **lateral and medial epicondyles**, which are the rounded protrusions of the humerus.

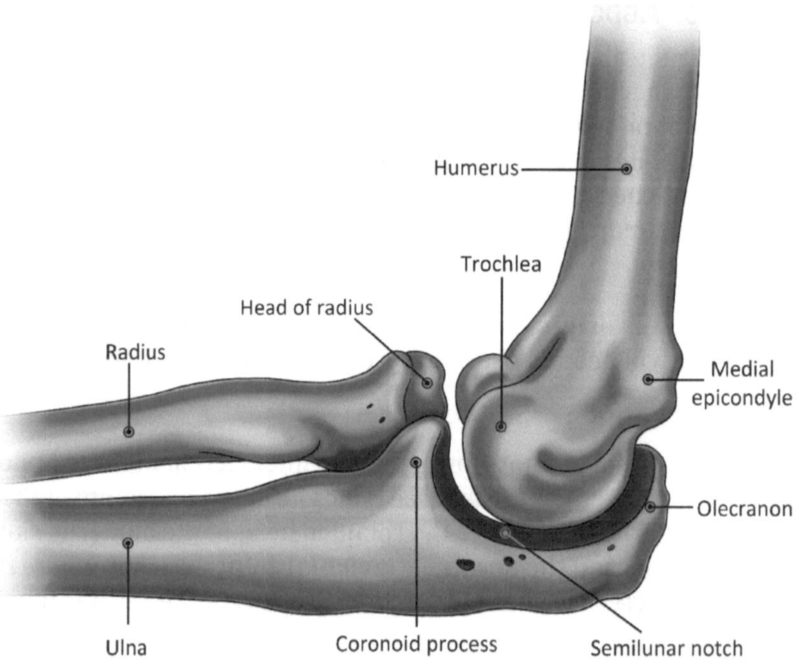

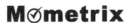

Coding Procedures of Arm and Wrist

Codes in this section refer to the shafts and distal ends of the **radius** (the thinner forearm bone) and the **ulna** (the thicker, longer forearm bone). These two bones form the forearm, which is then linked to the **wrist**. The wrist is a complex joint, made up of eight **carpal bones** and the associated connective tissue, which bridges the space between the forearm and the rest of the hand. Although there are several carpal bones, several procedures focus on the **scaphoid** and **lunate** bones, particularly when it comes to fractures. This is because those two bones are the closest to the forearm and are more likely to be damaged or fractured.

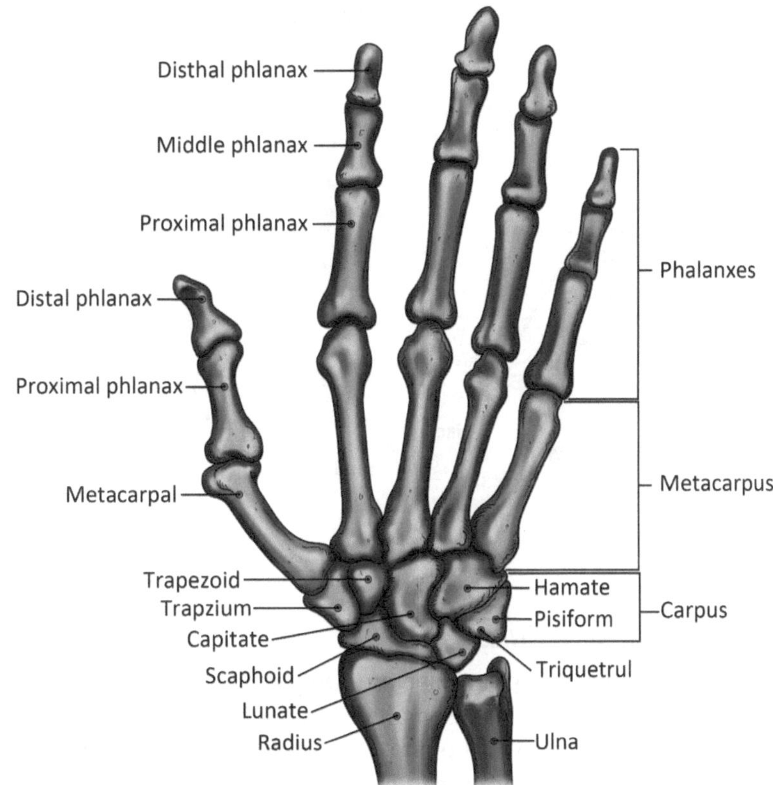

Coding Procedures of Hand and Fingers

Procedures listed in this section cover the structures of the hand. Working from the proximal end of the hand at the wrist, there are the **metacarpals**, a set of five bones that link to the wrist and form the basis for the fingers. From the metacarpals, we move into the **phalanges**, which form the actual fingers. There are 14 phalanges in total: three for each finger and two for the thumb. The phalanges are divided into the **proximal**, **middle**, and **distal phalanges**, the last of which carries the fingernail.

In terms of soft tissues, there are various muscles and tendons that allow the fingers to move and grip; and various joints, such as the **metacarpophalangeal** (metacarpal bones to phalanges) and **interphalangeal** (between the phalanges) joints.

Coding Procedures of Pelvis and Hip

Procedures listed in this section cover the **pelvis**, the lowest part of the trunk. Similar to the shoulders, the pelvis is made up of multiple interlocking bones. Three bones form the ring-like structure of the pelvis, starting posteriorly with the **sacrum**, which links with the **coccyx** (tailbone) and connects to the spinal column. On either side of the sacrum are the **hip bones**, the large, curved bones made up of three portions: the **ilium** (the wing-like crest), the **ischium** (the lower curved portion), and the **pubis** (the anterior curved portion that connects the hip bones together). These bones are important for supporting the body's weight and protecting the various organs of the lower body.

The pelvis is also the site of the **hip joint**, which is the ball-and-socket joint formed by the bowl-shaped socket in the hip bones called the **acetabulum**; and the rounded head of the femur. Other major joints covered by procedures in this section include the **sacroiliac**, the joint between the sacrum and the ilium of the hip bone; and the **symphysis pubis**, the joint between the pubis portion of the hip bones.

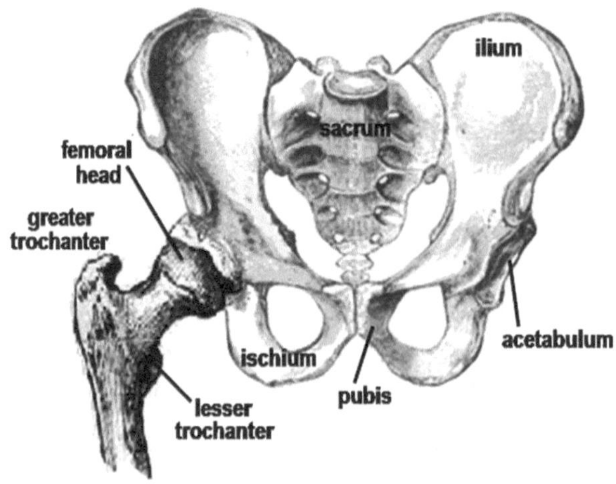

Leg

Coding Procedures of Thigh and Knee

The section covering the region of the upper leg commonly called the **thigh** is taken up by the **femur**, the long, thick bone that connects proximally to the pelvis and distally to the tibia and the lower leg. The femur is the longest bone of the body and consists of the **shaft**, or the long central piece; and the two rounded **epiphyses**, or extremities.

This section also includes the **knee**, a major hinge joint that is formed at the connection between the femur and the bones of the lower leg, particularly the tibia. The knee also includes the **patella**, the shield-like bone that forms the kneecap. Several codes also deal with the major joints of the knee, including the **tibiofemoral joint**, located between the femur and the tibia; the **patellofemoral joint**, located between the femur and the patella; and also the **meniscus**, or the jelly-like pad of connective tissue within the knee proper.

Coding Procedures of Lower Leg and Ankle

The lower portion of the leg consists of two bones: the **tibia,** the thicker anterior medial bone that forms the **shin**; and the **fibula**, the thinner posterior lateral bone. These two bones function in a similar fashion to the radius and ulna, but they connect the knee to the ankle.

The **ankle** joint links the bones of the lower leg to the bones of the foot, specifically the **talus**. The ankle is made up of the **talocrural joint** between the talus and the tibia and fibula, the **subtalar joint** between the talus and the calcaneus, and the **inferior tibiofibular joint** between the tibia and the fibula at the lower portion. In addition to these major joints, several codes address procedures involving the **Achilles tendon,** the major tendon that runs along the back of the leg and the foot.

CODING PROCEDURES OF THE FEET AND TOES

The feet and toes are the most **inferior** (anatomically lowest) portion of the body. The feet and toes are similar in structure to the hand and wrist and are capable of similar movement. Moving from the proximal portion of the foot forward, there are seven **tarsal** bones: the **talus**; the **calcaneus**; the medial, intermediate, and lateral **cuneiforms**; the **cuboid**; and the **navicular.** These bones help to form and connect the ankle joint to the rest of the foot, with the calcaneus forming the heel of the foot.

Proceeding along are the five **metatarsals**, which function similar to the metacarpals of the hand and connect the toes to the rest of the foot. Much like the hand, the foot terminates into 14 **phalanges**: two in the big toe and three in each other toe. Much like procedures of the hand, procedures of the foot cover treatment of several joints, such as the **metatarsophalangeal joint**, located between the metatarsals and the phalanges; and also soft tissue such as the **plantar fascia**, the connective tissue for the muscles on the bottom of the foot.

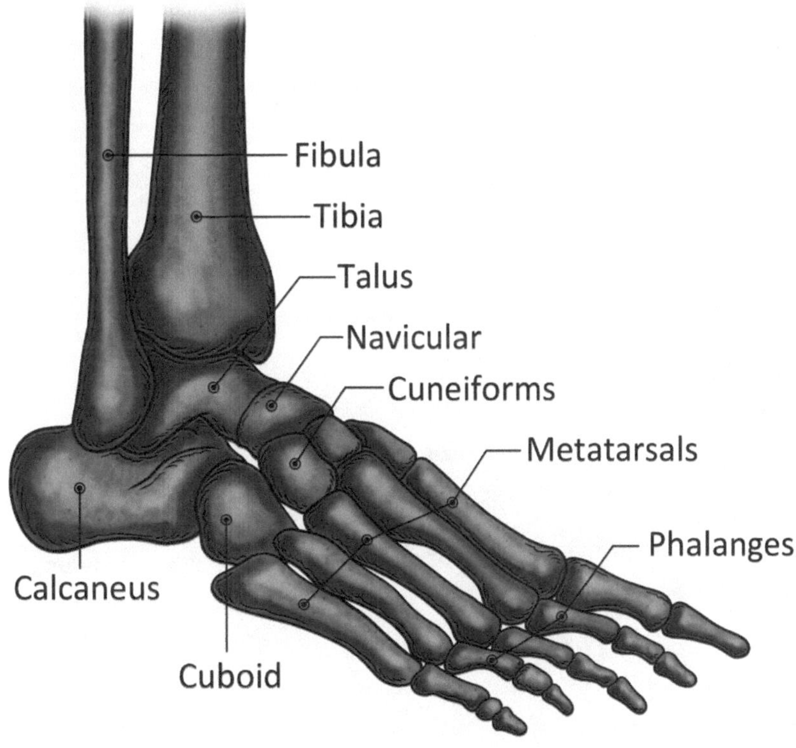

Respiratory System

Anatomical Structures and Procedures

The respiratory system consists of the organs that provide oxygen to the rest of the body via breathing. Important structures involved in this section include the following:

- The **nose** and the accessory **sinuses**
- The **larynx**, or voice box
- The **trachea**, the main tube that leads to the lungs, and the **bronchi** that branch off of it
- The **lungs**, in which oxygen and carbon dioxide are exchanged and the blood is oxygenated; and the **pleura**, the membrane surrounding the lungs

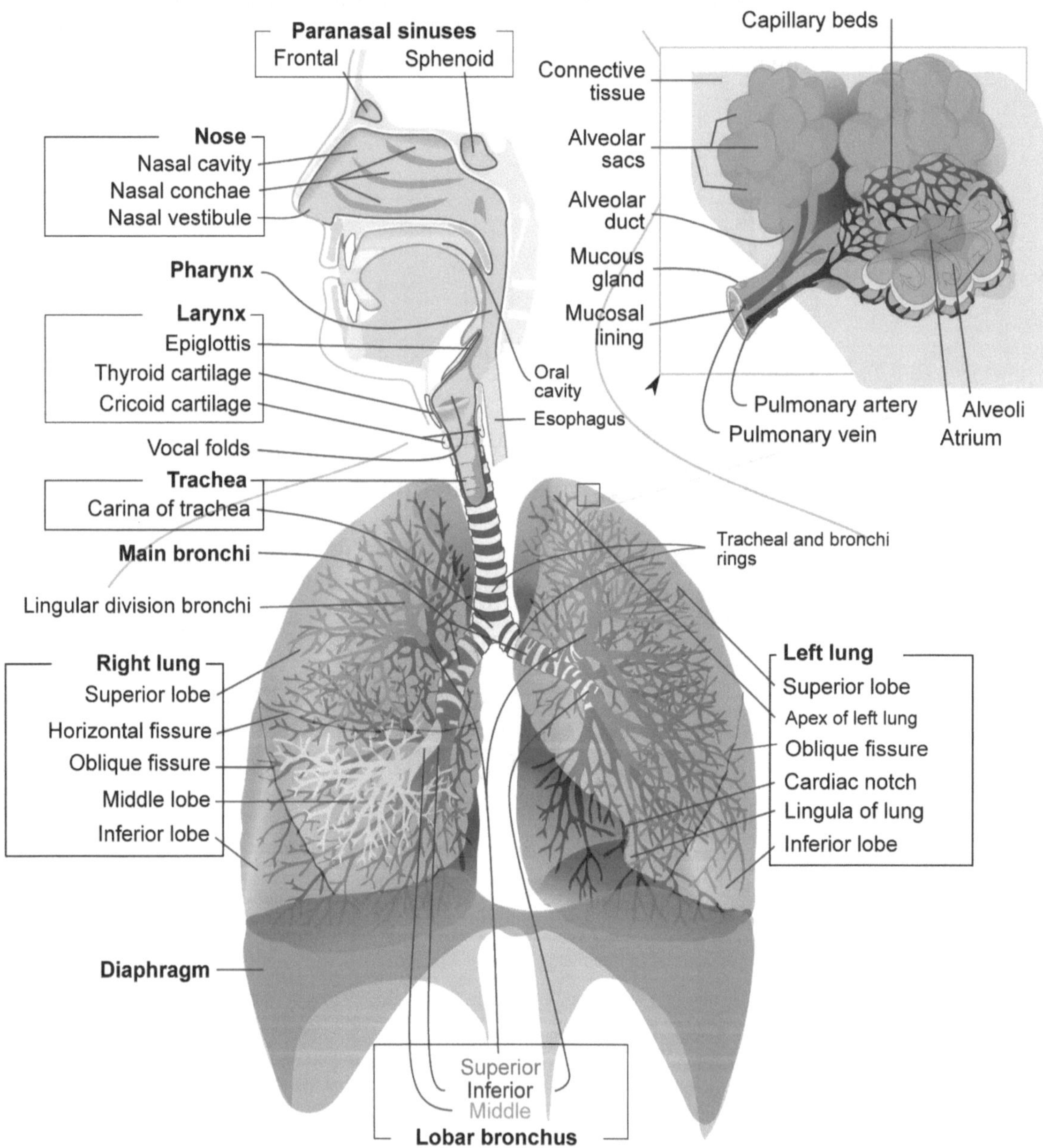

This section in CPT covers codes **30000** through **32999**, which include the following types of procedures:

- Incision, excision, introduction, repair, and destruction of tissues of the nose, larynx, trachea, bronchi, and lungs
- Endoscopies of the sinuses, larynx, trachea, bronchi, and lungs
- Video-assisted thoracic surgery of the lungs
- Lung transplants
- Therapeutic treatments of the lung, such as stereotactic radiation therapy and surgical collapse therapy

Video-Assisted Thoracic Surgery and Related Procedures

Video-assisted thoracic surgery is a type of endoscopic surgery used for correcting issues of the **thorax** (chest). When a video-assisted thoracic surgery is performed, a flexible tube with a mounted light and camera, called an **endoscope**, is inserted through the thoracic cavity in order to directly inspect the lungs and allow surgical tools access without performing a more invasive procedure. Endoscopic procedures involving the thorax (especially the lungs) are also referred to as **thoracoscopies**.

A video-assisted thoracic surgery, particularly in this section, is performed for a variety of reasons, including the following:

- Biopsies of lung tissue and pleura
- Surgical excision of lesions on the lungs and pleura
- Removal or resection of lung, pleura, or lymph tissue
- Removal of excess fluid or air from the pleural area

Cardiovascular System

Anatomical Structures and Procedures

The cardiovascular system consists of the organs and systems that circulate blood, fluid, nutrients, and other substances throughout the body. It also removes waste products for disposal. Structures involved in this section include the following:

- The **heart**, the muscular pump that drives the system
- The pericardium, a protective sac that reduces friction between the heart and organs within the mediastinum
- The **blood vessels**, which are divided into **arteries** that take blood away from the heart and **veins** that carry blood to the heart

The cardiovascular system is covered by codes **33016** through **37799**, including the following procedures:

- Treatment and repair of conditions involving the heart and **pericardium** (heart membrane)
- Implanting devices, including defibrillators, monitors, and prosthetics
- Heart transplants
- Blood vessel repair and reconstruction
- Treatment of **aneurysms** (enlargements of artery wall) and **thromboses** (blood clots inside a blood vessel)
- Blood vessel grafting and transposition
- Preparation for and execution of **hemodialysis** (artificial filtering of waste from the blood)

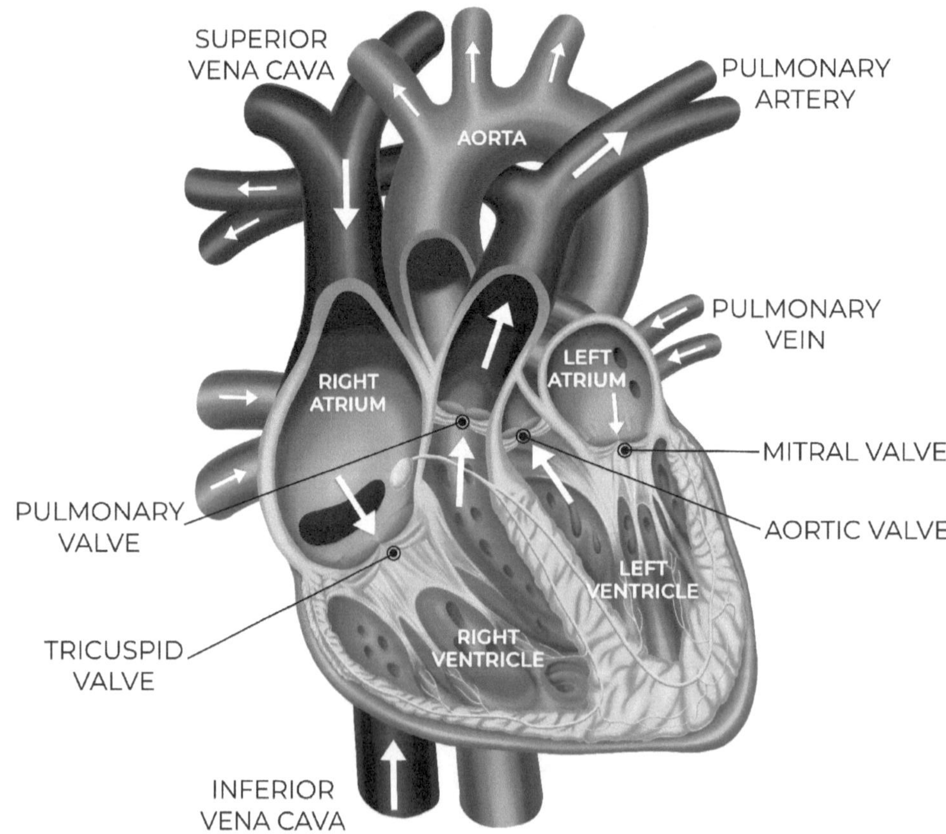

PACEMAKER AND DEFIBRILLATOR PLACEMENT

Pacemakers, which help control abnormal heart rhythms, and **defibrillators**, which restore the heartbeat with an electrical shock, are common implants meant to treat heart conditions. When coding for these procedures, there are several factors that can influence the code required, including the following:

- The type of device (temporary pacemaker, implanted pacemaker, implanted defibrillator, etc.)
- Whether it is a new or replacement device (such as an upgrade from an older device) or the removal of a device
- The number of leads on the device (single, dual, or multiple leads)
- The method of insertion, such as via a thoracotomy or transcatheter

Codes in this section also cover the repositioning of existing devices as well. Unless otherwise noted, the codes should also indicate the surgical procedures needed to insert or remove the device.

CABG

A coronary artery bypass graft (CABG) is a procedure in which blood vessels from other portions of the body are grafted to the heart and major vessels (the **aorta** and the **vena cava**) to allow for blood flow to reach tissues of the heart, typically due to poor or obstructed flow in the existing vessels.

There are two factors that must be considered when coding for a CABG. The first is the **type of graft** that is being used, because that is what forms the initial categorization: **venous grafting** (in which veins are used), **arterial grafting** (in which arteries are used), or **combined arterial-venous grafting** (in which both types of tissue are used). When coding a combined grafting, the codes in the "Arterial Grafting" section (codes **33533** through **33536**) are used as the primary codes because the codes in the "Combined" section (**33517** through **33523**) are add-on codes. The second factor to consider is the number of grafts being used, which range from one to four or more.

BYPASS GRAFTS OF BLOOD VESSELS

Bypass grafts are used to reroute blood around obstructions in a blood vessel. Typically, this is done by taking a portion of a blood vessel from another part of the body and transplanting it to the affected site, allowing blood flow to bypass the obstruction.

Much like when coding CABGs, there are certain factors that must be accounted for when coding bypass grafts. To begin with, check the **type of graft** being used. Possibilities include a venous graft, an **in situ vein** (rerouting through an existing vein), an arterial graft, or a **composite graft** (made of multiple different segments linked together). The other major factor is the **sites being linked**, such as a carotid-vertebral bypass, which determines the primary code. This section also includes add-on codes for the harvest of certain vessels for grafting procedures.

VENOUS AND ARTERIAL ORDERS

When coding certain cardiovascular procedures, such as **angiographies** (inspections of a blood vessel via a catheter), there will be mentions of "orders" of veins or arteries. **Orders** are a method of categorizing particular arteries or veins depending on their position in a grouping, known as a **vascular family.**

The best way to describe orders is to think of them like off-ramps of a highway. Each order is one "turnoff" away from the respective major vessels, the **aorta** and the **vena cava**. Thus, the **first**

order is a branch off the major vessel, the **second order** is a branch off the first order, and so on. When coding a procedure involving orders, check what order the mentioned artery or vein is in the procedure description.

Refer to "Vascular Families for Interventional Radiology Coding" in the appendices section of the CPT codebook to clarify the orders within the arterial and venous vascular family.

Hemic and Lymphatic

Anatomical Structures and Procedures

The hemic and lymphatic system consists of the organs and tissues that help filter, maintain, and protect the body's blood supply. Procedures coded in this section include the following anatomical structures:

- The **spleen**, which filters the blood and removes dead or diseased cells
- **Bone marrow**, the spongy tissue inside bones that produces new blood cells
- **Stem cells**, undifferentiated cells used for repairing and building tissue
- The **lymph nodes**, nodules of tissue that filter **lymph fluid** and contain white blood cells
- The **lymph channels**, which circulate lymph fluid throughout the body

Procedures involving the hemic and lymphatic systems are covered by codes **38100** through **38999** and include the following:

- Excision, repair, and laparoscopy of the spleen
- Procedures involving bone marrow or stem cells
- Transplant procedures
- Incision, excision, removal, and introduction of lymph nodes and related tissues

Mediastinum and Diaphragm

Anatomical Structures and Procedures

This section covers two separate anatomical structures: the mediastinum and the diaphragm. The **mediastinum** is the term used for the compartment that makes up the **thoracic cavity** and contains the heart and its vessels; esophagus; trachea; and all associated nerves, muscles, and lymph nodes. The mediastinum is bordered on the sides by the lungs and at the bottom by the diaphragm. The **diaphragm** is a sheet of skeletal muscle that stretches across the bottom of the thoracic cavity like a floor. The diaphragm not only separates the thoracic cavity, it also contracts and expands to draw air into the lungs.

Procedures involving the mediastinum and the diaphragm are covered by codes **39000** through **39599** and include the following:

- Incision, excision, and resection on the mediastinum
- Endoscopy procedures on the mediastinum
- Repair of the diaphragm

Digestive System

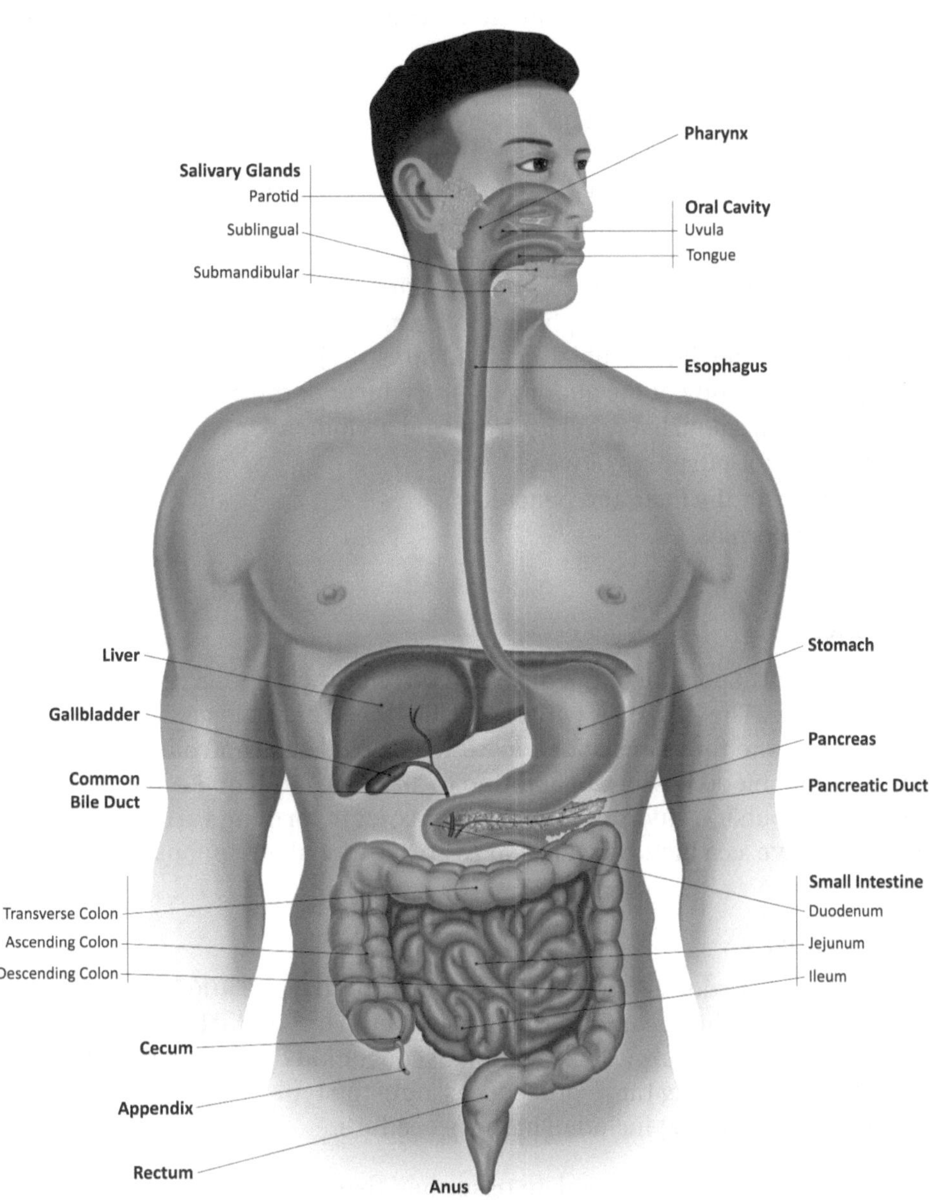

ANATOMICAL STRUCTURES

The digestive system consists of a series of interlinked organs and associated systems that intake and digest nutrients, breaking them down to a form usable by the body, and then excrete any remaining waste matter. Digestion begins when nutrients are taken into the mouth and past the lips, and are chewed before being swallowed. The mouth contains the **tongue**; **dentoalveolar structures** such as the teeth; the **palate**, which forms the roof of the mouth and the dangling **uvula**; as well as **salivary glands and ducts.** Proceeding down from the mouth, food passes through the **pharynx**, down the **esophagus**, and into the **stomach**. It then passes through the stomach to the

duodenum, as various enzymes from the **liver**, **gallbladder**, and **pancreas** are added to the mix. Food then passes through the rest of the **small intestine** (the **jejunum** and the **ileum**) before passing over the **appendix** and into the **large intestine**—made up of the **ascending**, **transverse**, and **sigmoid colons**—before waste is stored in the **rectum** and expelled through the **anus.**

PROCEDURES

Procedures involving the digestive system are covered by CPT codes **40490** through **49999**, which are divided into related headings and subheadings throughout the section. Codes are grouped together based on the anatomical location of the procedure taking place. Procedures in this section include the following:

- Incision, excision, and repair of various bodily structures
- Endoscopic investigation of the esophagus, intestines, colon, anus, and **biliary tract** (the connection between the liver, gallbladder, and intestine)
- **Laparoscopic** (endoscopy of the abdomen) procedures of the esophagus, stomach, intestines, appendix, colon, liver, biliary tract, and abdomen
- **Bariatric surgery** for purposes of weight loss
- Transplant surgery of the liver and pancreas
- Surgical repair of hernias

LIPS

ANATOMICAL PURPOSE

The lips are the most external portion of the digestive system, and they serve as the primary opening for nutrient intake. The lips meet with the rest of the skin of the face at a point referred to as the **vermilion border**, and they consist of two fleshy protrusions controlled by facial muscles and containing nerves and blood vessels. In addition to allowing food intake and protecting the oral cavity and teeth from the outside environment, the lips assist in forming various speech sounds and facial expressions and serve as a tactile organ, and as an additional erogenous zone due to their sensitivity.

CHEILOPLASTY PROCEDURES

Cheiloplasty procedures (CPT codes 40700–40702, 40720, 40761, and 40650–40654) refer to surgical procedures involving the repair and restoration of the lips. In CPT, cheiloplasty codes cover plastic surgery of the lips and the surgical correction of congenital **cleft lip**, a deformity that creates a split in the upper lip. When coding these procedures, note the type and purpose of the repair as well as the number of stages (if any) included in the procedure.

These codes are only for repairing the actual lip tissue and fixing cleft lips. Other reconstructive procedures will use codes from the integumentary system and are noted under the codes in this section.

MOUTH

ANATOMICAL STRUCTURES

The mouth is divided into two sections: the vestibule of the mouth and the oral cavity. The **vestibule of the mouth** is made up of all the parts outside of the dentoalveolar structures: the inner tissue of the cheeks and lips, the mucosal and submucosal portions thereof, and the space between them and the teeth. The **oral cavity** itself contains the teeth; gums; tongue; and the **floor of the mouth,** which is the fleshy tissue underneath the tongue. Because much of the mouth's interior consists of soft tissue, many of the procedure codes relating to it describe lesion or mass removal and the repair of any damage stemming from trauma or defects.

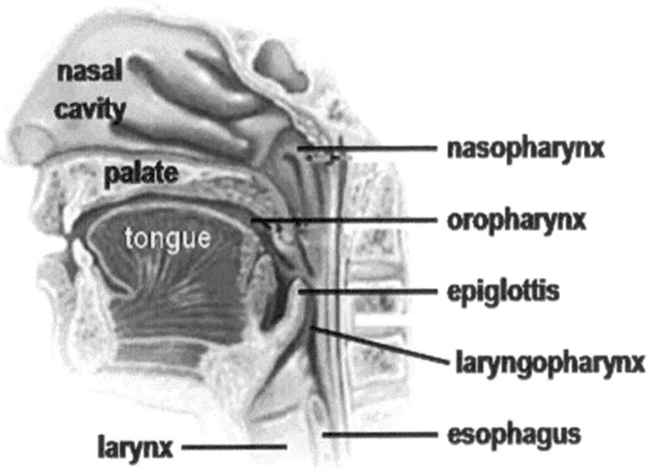

Dentoalveolar Structures

Dentoalveolar structures are the structures including and surrounding the teeth, **gingiva** (the gums), and associated structures such as the **alveolar process** (the bony sockets that hold the teeth). These structures are designed to chew and tear through food, allowing it to be digested easily and increase its exposure to saliva.

Most of the codes in this section cover the excision of lesions or foreign bodies from the soft tissue and repair of gum tissues and both soft and bony portions of the alveolar process. These codes do not involve actual dental procedures, only surgical ones; dental procedures are described in a completely separate text.

Palate and Uvula

The **palate** is the bone and tissue that form the roof of the mouth, separating the oral cavity from the nasal cavity above it. The palate consists of a layer of mucosal and soft tissue (the **soft palate**) that covers the harder bone (the **hard palate**) just above. Codes involving the palate typically refer to destruction of soft tissue and masses and the repair of a **cleft palate**, which is an opening (typically congenital) in the palate.

The **uvula** (also known as the palatine uvula) is the downward-hanging flap of tissue located near the back of the mouth. In addition to helping produce saliva, the uvula helps to close off and prevent food from entering the **nasopharynx**, the opening that leads to the nasal cavity. Codes involving the uvula involve drainage of abscesses, excision or destruction of lesions, and the removal of the uvula itself.

Salivary Glands and Ducts

The **salivary glands** are specialized glands located in the mouth that produce **saliva**, a fluid that helps lubricate food while it is chewed. In addition to hundreds of minor salivary glands, the mouth has three pairs of major salivary glands: the **parotid** (on the side of the face behind the jaw), **submandibular** (below the jaw), and **sublingual** (below the tongue) glands. Saliva is carried from the glands to the mouth via **salivary ducts**.

This section deals mostly with soft tissue, which is reflected by the procedures listed. Most of the codes in this section involve the treatment of abscesses; the excision of cysts, tumors, and glands; and the repair of salivary ducts.

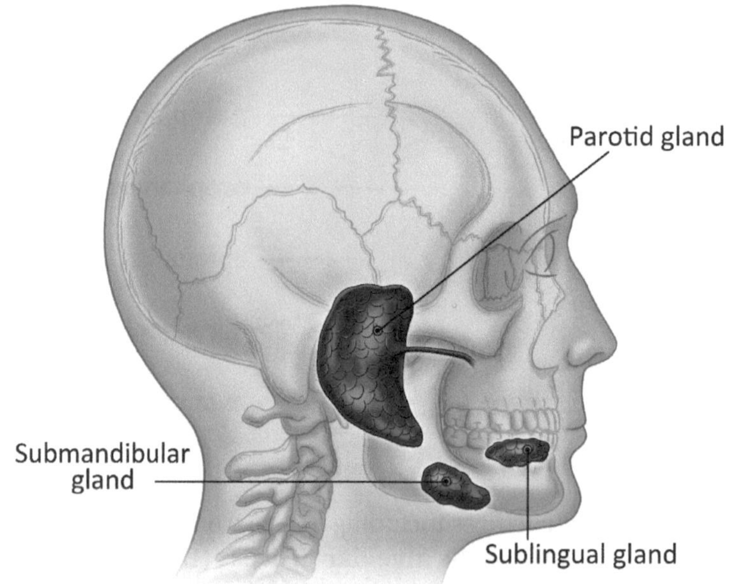

Salivary Glands

Pharynx, Adenoids, and Tonsils

The **pharynx** is the chamber located directly behind the mouth, which connects the mouth and nasal cavities to the esophagus and larynx. In addition to serving as a point of connection, the pharynx helps with speech.

The **adenoids** and **tonsils** are part of the lymphatic system located in the pharynx. The adenoids are located behind and on either side of the uvula on the roof of the pharynx, whereas the tonsils are located at the rear of the pharynx inside the lateral walls and behind the tongue. The adenoids and tonsils help to capture and eliminate inhaled and ingested bacteria.

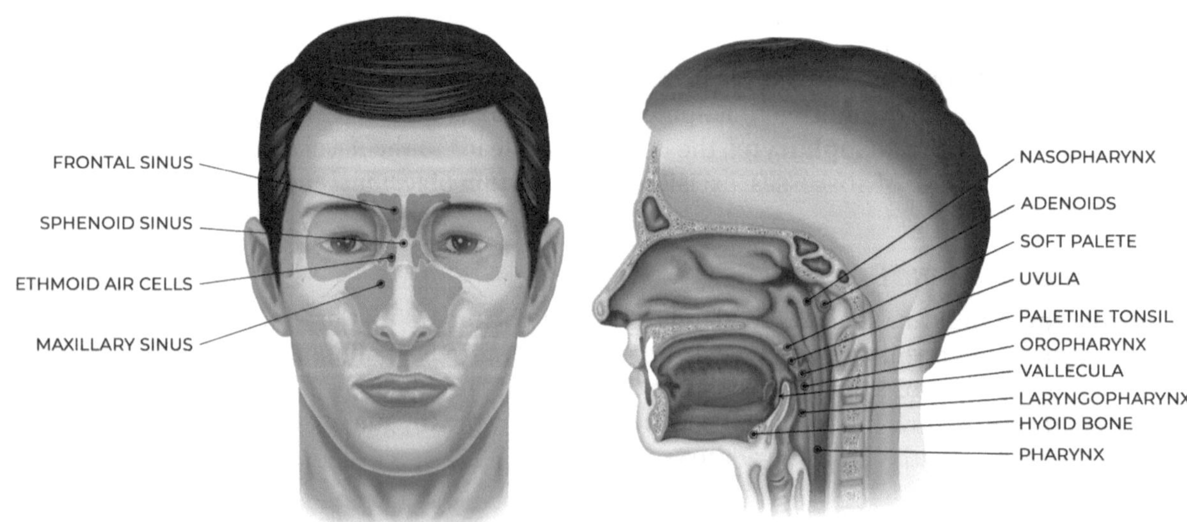

Tonsillectomy and Adenoidectomy Procedures

Tonsillectomies and adenoidectomies (CPT codes 42820–42845) are the surgical removal of the tonsils and adenoids, typically due to chronic infection or obstruction of the esophagus or larynx. Although this is typically done on patients under the age of 12, it can also be performed on adults. When coding these procedures, there are several factors that must be taken into account when selecting the correct code. First, check **what is being removed**, whether it is the tonsils, the adenoids, or both. Second, check the **patient's age**. The code may differ depending on whether the patient is a child or adult. Finally, check if this is a **radical resection**, which involves the removal of the tonsils and adjacent tissues, cells, and/or lymph nodes.

Esophagus

The esophagus is a tube of fibrous and muscular tissue that connects the pharynx to the stomach. The esophagus runs down behind the heart through the mediastinum and the diaphragm before connecting to the uppermost part of the stomach. Food is passed down the esophagus via muscular contractions, and a pair of **sphincters** (muscular gates) prevent food and stomach contents from flowing back toward the mouth.

Procedures involving the esophagus include excision of masses and tissue, endoscopic procedures of the esophagus and passing through it, laparoscopic procedures of the esophagus and the upper portion of the stomach, repair procedures (including the insertion of prosthetics), and manipulation of the esophageal structure.

Endoscopic Procedures

The esophagus is involved in a variety of endoscopic procedures due to its easy access via the mouth and its connection to the stomach. The procedures listed in this section are divided into three types: **esophagoscopy**, or endoscopic inspection and procedures of the esophagus itself; **esophagogastroduodenoscopy**, which is an endoscopic procedure involving the gastrointestinal tract from the esophagus, through the stomach, and into the duodenum; and **endoscopic retrograde cholangiopancreatography** (ERCP), a combination of endoscopy and fluoroscopy used to diagnose and treat issues of the pancreatic and biliary ducts.

There are several important factors to take into consideration when coding these procedures. For esophagoscopies, check the **point of entry** (oral or nasal), the **type of scope** (rigid or flexible), and **any additional procedures** (biopsy, removal of lesions, dilation, etc.). For **esophagogastroduodenoscopies**, check which **procedures** are performed (e.g., removal of foreign bodies, injections). Finally, **ERCP** is always performed with another procedure—for example, an ERCP with biopsy, or an ERCP with collection of a specimen by brushing or washing. In addition, many of the procedure codes come with a list of even more codes that are not to be reported alongside them (e.g., do not report 43263 in conjunction with 43260).

Stomach

Anatomy and Procedures

The stomach is a hollow, flexible, muscular organ that rests in the left upper quadrant of the abdomen and connects to the esophagus and the small intestine. The stomach can be separated into four sections: the **cardia**, which connects to the esophagus; the **fundus**, or upper curved portion; the **body**, which makes up the central region of the stomach; and the **pylorus**, which connects to the small intestine at the duodenum. The stomach's purpose is to break down chewed food for digestion via the secretion of enzymes and acid.

Procedures involving the stomach include gastrotomy, surgical removal of tissues, laparoscopic procedures, **gastric intubation** (insertion of a tube into the stomach via the nose or mouth), **bariatric surgery** (surgery involving the stomach and portions of the small intestine), and the insertion or removal of implanted devices.

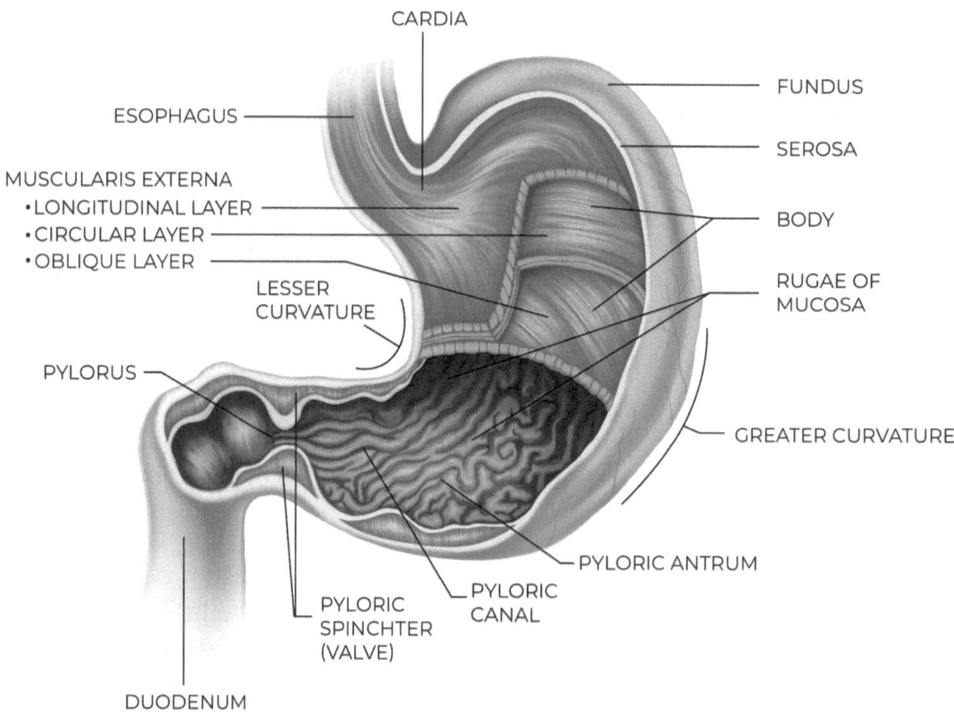

Gastric Bypass Procedures

Gastric bypass procedures (CPT codes 43770–43775) are surgical procedures in which a large portion of the stomach is surgically bypassed, leaving a smaller pouch that is connected to the small intestine. This is typically done to treat morbid obesity and related conditions. Gastric bypass procedures are included in a variety of codes in this section, mostly for procedures meant to treat obesity. When coding these sorts of procedures, check if the procedure notes mention a **Roux-en-Y gastroenterostomy**. A Roux-en-Y procedure is a specific procedure in which the small intestine is divided and rearranged into a Y shape and connected to the stomach. Procedures that use the Roux-en-Y approach require different codes than standard bypass procedures.

Intestines

Anatomy

The intestines are long, hollow muscular organs that aid digestion by extracting nutrients from digested food and by moving solid waste toward the rectum and anus for excretion. The intestines are made up of two distinct organs.

The first is the **small intestine**, which handles most of the absorption. The small intestine is divided into three distinct regions: the **duodenum**, which connects to the stomach; the **jejunum**, which makes up the upper portion; and the **ileum**, the bottom portion that connects to the large intestine.

The second is the **large intestine**, which helps extract water and salt and moves solid waste to the end of the digestive tract. The large intestine can be divided into six sections: the **cecum**, which connects the large intestine to the end of the small intestine; the **ascending colon**, which moves waste upward; the **transverse colon**, which goes across the upper part of the abdomen; the **descending colon**; and the **sigmoid colon**, which connects to the **rectum**.

Colectomy

A colectomy is a surgical procedure involving the removal of part or all of the large intestine for the purpose of treating diseases or ongoing issues. Colectomy procedures are surgical, and they can be done either openly or via a laparoscopic approach. There are several factors that must be accounted for when a colectomy procedure is coded. The first matter is whether the colectomy is done **surgically or via a laparoscope**. Next, check whether the procedure is **partial or total**, meaning whether part or all of the large intestine is removed. Finally, consider what **other procedures** are performed with the colectomy, such as a **colostomy** (connecting the colon to an opening in the body) or an **anastomosis** (connecting two parts of the colon together).

Stomal Endoscopy

A **colonoscopy through a stoma,** or stomal endoscopy, is when an endoscopic procedure enters the intestine through a **stoma,** an artificially created opening in the body. In this case, the stoma is typically a percutaneous opening from the colon to the outside of the body, or a **colostomy.** These procedures involve examination or treatment through the ileum and all the way to the cecum.

There are several factors to take into account when coding these procedures. In particular, attention should be paid to the **location being studied** (i.e., the ileum or the entire colon). Next, pay attention to what, if any, additional procedures are performed during the procedure.

Colonoscopies other than through a stoma can be found in the "Rectum" heading of CPT.

Appendix

The appendix is a small, tube-like organ that protrudes just below the cecum located in the lower right quadrant of the abdomen. The appendix functions as a reservoir for beneficial gut bacteria, and it serves as part of the immune and lymphatic systems.

Procedures involving the appendix almost entirely revolve around its removal, typically related to appendicitis, which can be life-threatening if not treated promptly. Removal of the appendix can be performed surgically or laparoscopically. However, an appendectomy is not reported when it is incidental to another intra-abdominal surgical procedure. If it is medically necessary to remove the appendix during another intra-abdominal surgical procedure, use add-on code 44955 (Appendectomy; when done for indicated purpose at time of other major procedure).

Rectum

The rectum is the short, straightened end of the large intestine that connects the sigmoid colon to the anus. The rectum's purpose is to act as a storage site for fecal material received from the colon before it is expelled through the anus. Because of its location and connection to the anus, the rectum is a common entry point for some procedures seeking to access the intestines. Procedures involving the rectum include the removal of tumors and masses, surgical removal of portions of rectal tissue, colonoscopies, laparoscopic procedures, repair of damaged tissues, and manipulation of the anus and impacted fecal material.

COLONOSCOPIES

Colonoscopies are endoscopic procedures in which the endoscope enters the large intestine via the rectum for diagnostic or treatment purposes. This section deals with three distinct types of colonoscopy procedures, which vary based on how far the endoscope travels through the large intestine. A **proctosigmoidoscopy** is when the scope only examines the rectum and part of the sigmoid colon. A **sigmoidoscopy** is when the scope examines the entire rectum and sigmoid colon and may include part of the descending colon. A **colonoscopy** is when the entire large intestine, from rectum to cecum, is examined, and may include examination of the terminal ileum.

Colonoscopies can also include an examination through a stoma. Locate these codes by finding "Colonoscopy" in the index, followed by "Through stoma," and review the CPT code that most appropriately describes the procedure(s) performed. Codes will fall within the range of 44388 through 44408.

ANUS

The anus is the opening at the end of the digestive tract, completely opposite of the mouth. The purpose of the anus is to control the expulsion of **feces**, or solid waste products that are produced from the unwanted or unhealthy matter left over from digestion. The anus is the terminus of the large intestine and includes the **anal canal**, which is the open space between the **inner** and **outer anal sphincters**.

Procedures involving the anus include incisions for treatment of fistulas and perineal abscesses, excision of hemorrhoids, endoscopic procedures for tumor removal, repair of damage, and destruction of anal lesions.

HEMORRHOIDECTOMY

Procedures for the treatment of hemorrhoids, or swollen vascular structures in and around the anal canal, are covered in the "Anal" portion of the "Digestive" section. Treatment of this problem is typically done with a **hemorrhoidectomy**, or surgical removal of hemorrhoid tissue. When coding procedures involving the removal of hemorrhoids, pay attention to certain key factors in the procedure. First, check if the hemorrhoid being removed is **internal**, **external**, or **both**. If internal, check which **method** is being used, such as ligation or dearterialization. If external, or both internal and external, check on the **number of groups** that are being removed.

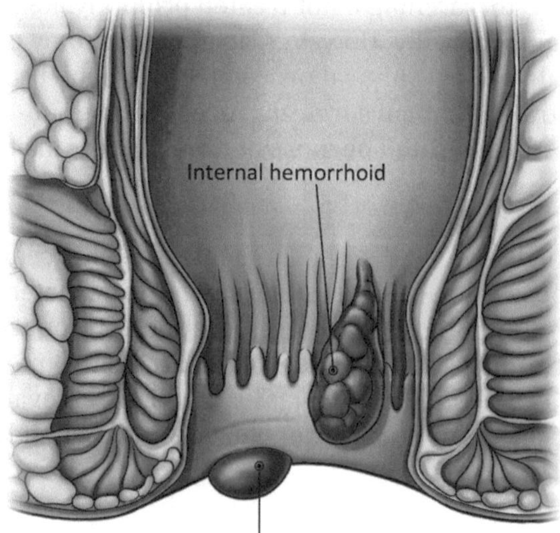

Liver

Anatomy and Procedures

The liver is a large, four-lobed organ that is located in the right upper quadrant of the abdomen. As an **accessory organ** (an organ that assists, but isn't directly involved) of the digestive system, the liver helps to metabolize carbohydrates, proteins, amino acids, and lipids; it breaks down many waste products and toxic substances such as alcohol; and it produces **bile**, a yellowish fluid that helps emulsify consumed fat. The liver is connected to the gallbladder and small intestine via the **common hepatic duct.**

Procedures involving the liver include biopsies, excisions, surgical removal of portions of the liver, transplants, repair of cysts and bleeding, laparoscopic treatments, and ablation of tumors through various methods.

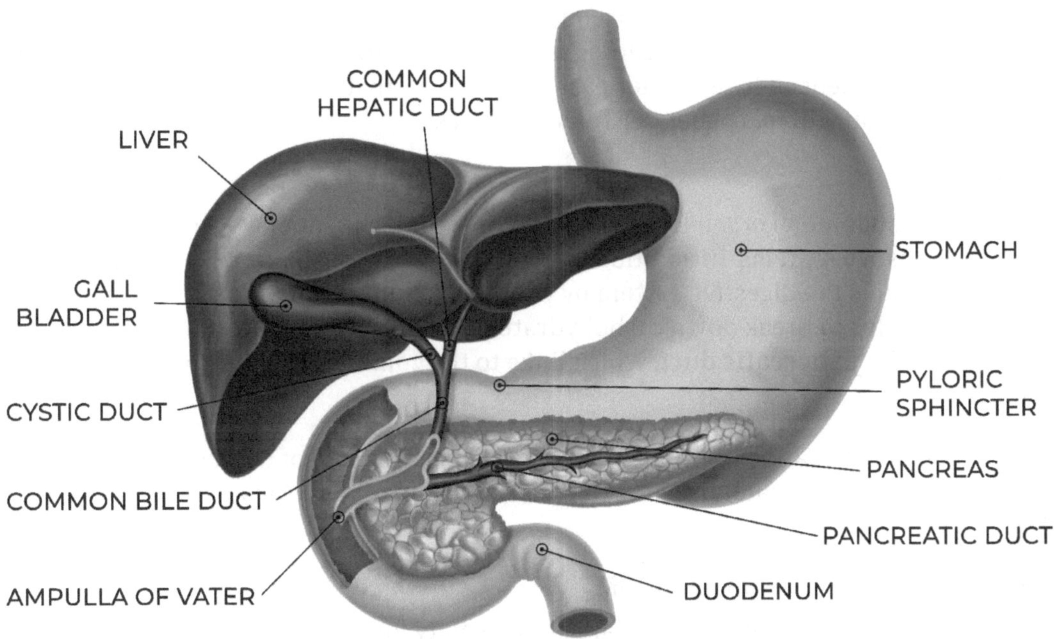

Liver Transplant

Liver transplants are a type of **allograft**, a graft or transplant that originates from a donor of the same species. Because the liver's numerous functions cannot be replicated with a prosthetic, a liver transplant is used to treat major issues such as acute liver failure. Liver transplant procedures require the careful consideration of several factors when reading the procedural notes in order to select the proper code. The first and major factor is the **source** of the transplanted tissue. If the source is from a living donor, then the actual removal of tissue, or **hepatectomy**, must be taken into account, as well as which **segments** of the liver are removed. If the source is from a cadaver, then the **backbench work**, or surgical removal and preparation, must be coded.

Biliary Tract

Anatomy and Procedures

The biliary tract (also called the **biliary system**) is a series of ducts and canals that connect the liver and gallbladder to the small intestine at the duodenum. The biliary tract is the path by which bile is transported from the liver into the small intestine. The **gallbladder** is included in this system because it is an accessory organ that stores bile when not in use. The biliary tract is made up of the **common hepatic duct**, into which the bile produced by the ducts and canals in the liver flows, which then joins the **cystic duct** from the gallbladder to form the **common bile duct**, which joins with the pancreatic duct and enters the small intestine through the **ampulla of Vater.**

Procedures in this section include the placement of catheters and stents, endoscopic and laparoscopic procedures, removal of the gallbladder, bile duct tumors, and cysts, and repair of the biliary tract's structures.

Exchange and Conversion Procedures Involving Biliary Tract Drains and Stents

The "Biliary Tract" section covers the placement of catheters and stents for the purposes of treatment. Biliary drainage catheters are used to drain bile out of the body when a bile duct is damaged or blocked, usually on a temporary basis. However, providers may decide to switch from a drain to a more permanent stent, depending on the duct's condition or the treatment plan. **Stents**, meanwhile, are flexible metal tubing or mesh designed to hold a duct open to correct blockages or aid in drainage, and they are meant to be used long term. When coding these exchanges, check the chart located in the "Biliary Tract" subheading in this section. In addition, several codes have their own separate code sequences, listed under each description, that note which codes shouldn't be reported in conjunction with placement or removal codes.

Pancreas

The pancreas is an abdominal organ located behind the stomach that plays an important role in the endocrine and digestive systems. In addition to producing a variety of important hormones for the body, the pancreas aids the digestive system by producing **pancreatic juice**, which neutralizes stomach acid and helps to break down carbohydrates, protein, and fat. The pancreas is linked to the small intestine via the **pancreatic duct,** which links to the common bile duct before it enters the ampulla of Vater.

Procedures involving the pancreas include biopsies, partial removal of the distal portion of the pancreas and the ampulla of Vater, repair of a pancreatic injury, and transplantation of a pancreatic allograft.

Abdomen, Peritoneum, and Omentum

The **abdomen**, or abdominal cavity, is the large body cavity located just below the thorax (or chest) and above the pelvis. The abdomen is an area that contains a variety of important organs, including the stomach, liver, intestines, gallbladder, pancreas, spleen, and kidneys. The upper boundary of the abdomen is formed by the diaphragm, whereas its floor is made up of the pelvic inlet.

The abdomen is enclosed by the **abdominal wall**, a three-layered wall of muscle that protects the organs inside and helps to maintain the body's shape. Just past the abdominal wall is the **peritoneum**, a large serous membrane that lines the inside of the abdominal cavity. The peritoneum is divided into two layers: the **parietal peritoneum**, which attaches to the abdominal wall; and the **visceral peritoneum**, which cushions and supports the various abdominal organs and their blood, lymph, and nervous connections. The peritoneum also includes the **greater and lesser omenta**, which enclose nerves, blood, lymph vessels, and connective tissue for the transverse colon and the curve of the stomach and the space between the stomach and liver, respectively.

Abdominal Hernia Repair

Hernias are abnormal exits or protrusions of an organ or organ tissue, such as intestines or the colon, through the wall of the cavity that contains it. The most common hernias involve the abdominal area, including the **groin**, which is the area where the abdomen ends and the legs begin.

Hernias are typically repaired surgically, and they often include the insertion of prosthetic mesh to repair the opening.

There are several factors to keep in mind when coding hernia repair procedures. These include the **patient's age** (because some hernias occur in younger patients), the **type of hernia** based on its location (such as inguinal or umbilical), whether the hernia is **initial or recurrent** (first time versus previously repaired), if the hernia is **incarcerated** (trapped) or **strangulated** (the blood flow is cut off), and the **method of repair** (such as surgical or laparoscopic).

The implantation of mesh or other prosthesis is included in all hernia repair codes and ranges from 49591 through 49596 and 49613 through 49618.

Urinary System

Anatomical Structures

The urinary system consists of a series of interlinked organs and vessels that eliminate fluid waste from the body in the form of **urine**. In doing so, the system helps to control the levels of electrolytes and metabolites in the body as well as regulating blood volume, pressure, and pH. The organs involved in this system are located in the abdomen and pelvis. Starting from the superior position, there are the **kidneys**, the bean-shaped organs that sit near the back of the abdominal cavity and filter the bloodstream. Wastes such as urea and uric acid then flow out of the kidneys through tubes of smooth muscle called **ureters**, which flow down into the **urinary bladder** located in the pelvic cavity. The bladder then stores urine until it is expelled through the **urethra**, another muscular tube that leads to the outside of the body.

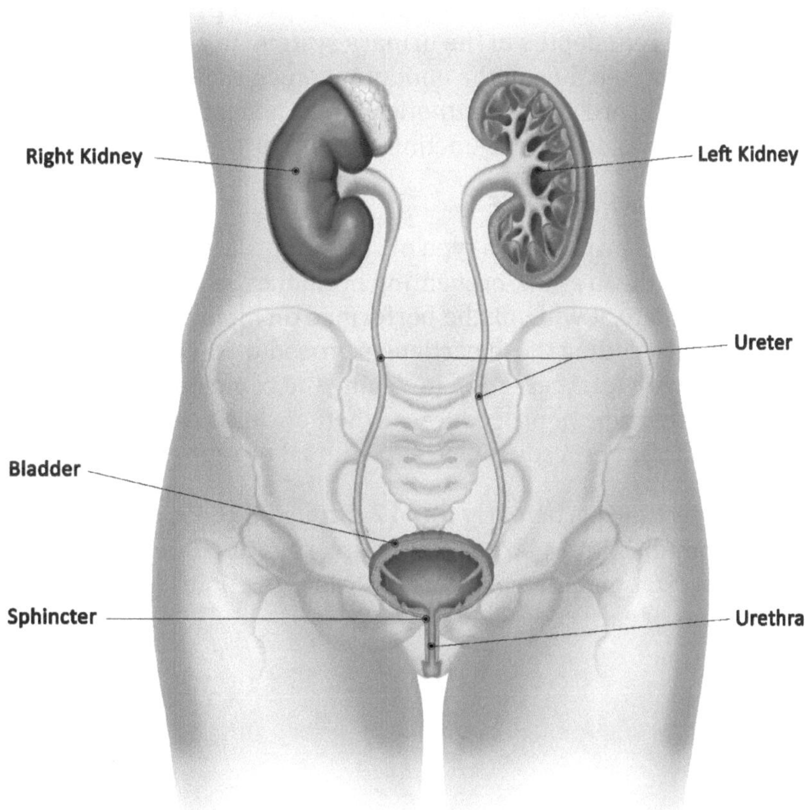

PROCEDURES

Procedures involving the urinary system are covered by codes **50010** through **53899** and are divided by anatomical location within the system. Procedures in this section include the following:

- Incision and excision of masses and lesions in the kidneys, ureter, bladder, and urethra
- Kidney transplants
- Introduction of substances and prosthetics into the system's structures
- Urodynamic procedures
- Repairing damaged tissue
- Laparoscopic procedures, including surgery
- Endoscopic procedures
- Transurethral surgical procedures
- Resection or destruction of prostate tissue
- Manipulation of the urethra for treatment purposes

It should be noted that, other than procedures involving the prostate, the procedures are identical regardless of the gender of the patient.

CYSTOSCOPY

Endoscopic procedures involving the urinary system (typically including the bladder) are usually referred to as cystoscopies. This section also includes **urethroscopies**, which include the urethra; as well as **cystourethroscopies**, which include the urethra, bladder, and ureter. These procedures cover diagnostic and surgical procedures involving the endoscopy. As always, diagnostic procedures are included in procedures meant for treatment.

When coding these procedures, it's important to note the **type of procedure** being performed because each one covers different depths of the urinary system. In addition, take note of the **additional procedures** performed during the endoscopy, such as insertions of stents or treatment of intrarenal strictures. Also, record any parenthetical notes beneath the procedure descriptions because some codes are not reported in conjunction with other codes.

TRANSURETHRAL RESECTION OF PROSTATE

A transurethral resection of the prostate is a type of surgical procedure used to remove or eliminate prostate tissue that obstructs the urethra, preventing normal expelling of urine. Because this is a procedure involving the prostate, it will only be performed on biologically male patients. There are a few factors to consider when coding these particular procedures. The first factor is whether it is a **partial or total resection**, with total resection involving the complete removal of the prostate. The second factor when coding this type of procedure is whether this is the initial encounter for the procedure or if this is a recurrent procedure to treat residual or regrown tissue.

Similar codes in the same section, particularly **52647** through **52649,** describe a transurethral resection of the prostate bundled into a larger procedure, such as a laser coagulation, laser enucleation, and laser vaporization of the prostate. Consider the notes listed in parentheses underneath the descriptions of each code.

Male Reproductive System

Anatomical Structures

The male reproductive system is made up of the sexual organs possessed by biologically male individuals. These organs are located in the pelvic region, and they are designed to assist in reproduction by producing semen and acting as erogenous zones. Semen production begins in the **testes**, which are suspended in an external, fleshy sac called the **scrotum**. Semen flows into the **epididymis**, where it is stored until use. Semen then flows through the **vas deferens**, or deferent duct, up and around until it joins with the **ejaculatory duct**. In the ejaculatory duct, the semen is mixed with fluid produced by the **seminal vesicle** and the **prostate** before being expressed into and through the urethra. The male urethra passes through the **penis**, the tube-shaped external reproductive and sexual organ.

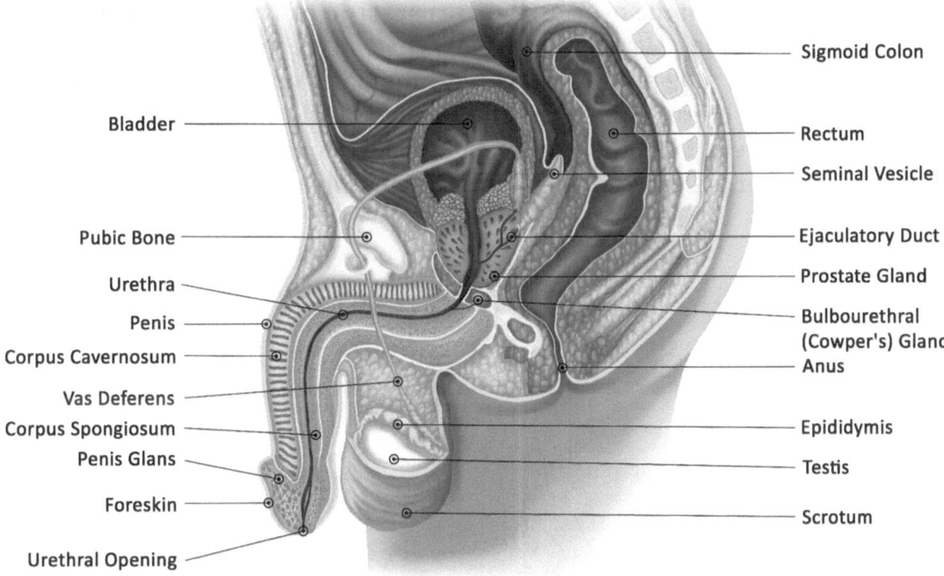

Circumcision

Circumcision is a type of excision procedure involving the surgical removal of the male **foreskin**. The foreskin is a double-layered fold of skin, muscle tissue, blood vessels, nerves, and mucous membrane that covers the penis and protects it from abrasion. Circumcision is typically performed at a very young age, often following birth, for cultural or religious reasons. In some cases, uncircumcised adults are circumcised due to medical necessity or during treatment for a related condition of the genitalia. Because of this, the **age of the patient** is a major factor when coding circumcision procedures: Most circumcision codes involve patients that are 28 days old or younger. In addition to age, the **method** of circumcision is also important. Note the method that is used and code appropriately.

Prostate Removal

The prostate is a gland located around the urethra just before the penis that produces fluid and constricts the portion of the urethra leading to the bladder during ejaculation. Prostate removal procedures, or **prostatectomies**, are performed in the event that the prostate becomes cancerous. There are several factors to take into account when selecting the proper codes for these procedures. The first factor is the **approach**, which is how the prostate is accessed during the procedure. The next factor to consider is the **level of removal**: whether the procedure is subtotal (partial) or radical (complete, including removal of additional tissue). Finally, make note of any **additional procedures**, such as lymph node biopsies, that are performed during the procedure. The procedure may automatically include certain other procedures, such as vasectomies, in the code. Included procedures should not be coded separately.

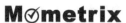

Female Reproductive System

Anatomical Structures

The female reproductive system is made up of the sexual organs possessed by biologically female individuals. These organs are in the pelvic region and assist in reproduction by producing eggs and carrying fertilized eggs to term, and they include erogenous zones. Starting from the organs involved in production, the system begins with the **ovaries**, which produce and store unfertilized eggs. These eggs are released from the ovaries and are captured by the **infundibulum**, the open, funnel-like portion of the **fallopian** (or uterine) **tubes.** The egg then moves down through the **ampulla** and into the fallopian tube proper before entering the **uterus**, the large, open organ where reproduction takes place. The uterus is linked to the **cervix** (the flexible, sphincter-like opening) by the **cervical canal.** Past the cervix lies the **vagina**, the tube-like opening that leads out of the body. The vagina then terminates at the external female sex organs, including the **vulva.**

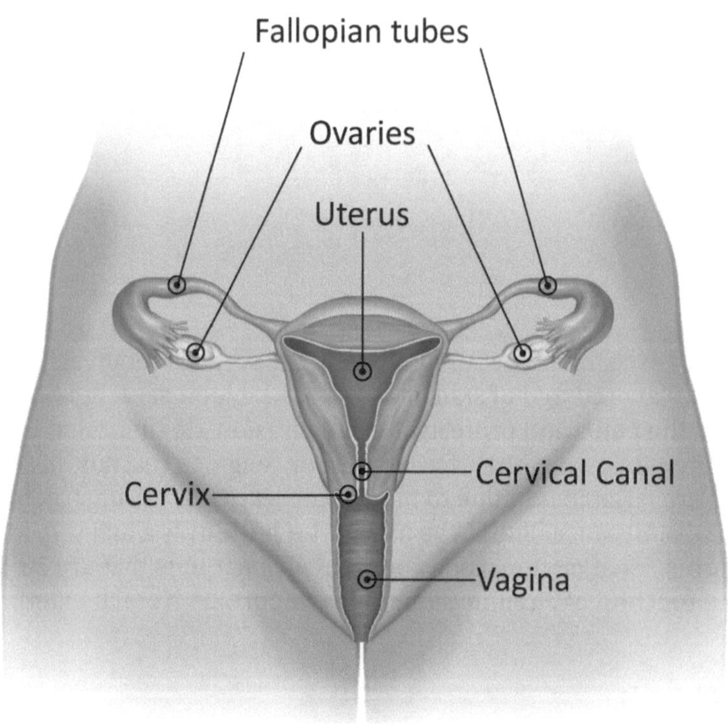

Excision Procedures of Vulva

When coding excision procedures of the vulva, or **vulvectomies**, it is important to recognize the common terms used when describing the procedures. There are four particular terms used when describing the procedures, which are defined as the following:

- **Simple** vulvectomy procedures involve the removal of benign or premalignant lesions in the skin and superficial subcutaneous tissue. These are the least intensive types of procedures.
- **Radical** vulvectomy procedures involve the removal of a malignancy in the skin, superficial tissue, and deeper subcutaneous tissue. During a radical vulvectomy, the lymph nodes and/or clitoris may also be removed.
- **Partial** vulvectomy procedures involve the removal of less than 80 percent of the benign or premalignant vulvar area.
- **Complete** vulvectomy procedures involve the removal of 80 percent or more of the vulvar area to treat any stage of malignant disease.

These codes are only for the actual removal procedures. Additional procedures, such as skin grafts or biopsies, will require additional codes.

Hysterectomy

A hysterectomy is a surgical procedure that involves the removal of the uterus, typically for therapeutic or treatment-related reasons. As with most intensive surgical procedures, it is important to read the procedural notes and consider several factors when coding them. The first is the **approach** of the surgery: whether the procedure is performed via a **supracervical** (an incision above the cervix) or **vaginal** (through the vaginal canal) approach. Also, check if the procedure is surgical or laparoscopic: Laparoscopic hysterectomy procedures are found in the "Laparoscopic" section. Next, check what **other structures** are removed, such as the vagina or ovaries. For vaginal approaches, the removal of additional structures is labeled under separate codes.

Maternity and Delivery

Most procedures involved in the "Maternity Care" section of CPT include **antepartum**, or prebirth, procedures and services. These procedures typically include prenatal history and examination, recording of the fetus's vital signs, routine urinalysis, and visits until the date of delivery. This section includes diagnostic and therapeutic **amniocentesis**, or extraction of amniotic fluid, as well as infusions and repair procedures.

The "Maternity Care" section also includes the treatment of **ectopic pregnancies**, which are when an otherwise viable fertilized egg implants outside of the uterus, such as on the ovary or inside the fallopian tube. These typically require surgical or laparoscopic intervention, and they often include relevant preparatory procedures.

Delivery

Procedures involving delivery, or the actual physical process of childbirth, are coded in multiple ways based on a number of factors. The first and most obvious one is the **method of delivery**. This covers traditional vaginal delivery (i.e., with no complications or intervention), as well as **Cesarean delivery**, which involves surgical intervention. Deliveries that occur after a previous Cesarean delivery are coded with different codes than a vaginal delivery.

Oftentimes, the code selection for delivery, antepartum, and postpartum care will depend on the type of insurance coverage the patient has. Some carriers only accept the **global obstetrical**

package, which bundles all three stages of pregnancy into one code (see CPT codes 59400, 59510, and 59610). In this case, a coder may report a code with no charges attached at the time of service, otherwise known as a **placeholder code** (0500F through 0503F), in order to keep a facility record that the patient was seen and what type of visit it was. On the other hand, other carriers or the circumstance surrounding the patient's pregnancy (e.g., they switch providers in the middle of treatment) may force a coder to report each stage of the pregnancy separately and at the time of service (see CPT codes 59409 through 59430, 59514, 59515, and 59612 through 59622).

Abortion

Abortion is a term used for the predelivery termination of a pregnancy. Abortions can be caused artificially by a provider or can result from bodily functions, trauma, or diseases (which are commonly referred to as **miscarriages**). Abortions discussed in CPT include the following:

- **Incomplete abortion**, in which some of the products of conception remain inside the body
- **Missed abortion**, in which the products of conception remain inside the body
- **Septic abortion**, resulting from an infection of the uterus
- **Induced abortion**, in which the abortion is caused by medical intervention

When coding abortion procedures, check the type of abortion, the **method of treatment**, and (in some cases) the **trimester** and **additional procedures**. For a complete spontaneous abortion, CPT guidelines advise reporting Hospital Services (CPT codes 99221 through 99233).

Endocrine System

Anatomical Structures

The endocrine system is a series of glands and organs that create and maintain multiple chemical reactions and feedback loops within the body. This is done by producing the necessary hormones for the body, which in turn regulate physiological, developmental, and behavioral processes. Major organs that are considered part of the endocrine system include the following:

- Thyroid glands, located in the neck on either side of the trachea
- Parathyroid glands, smaller glands attached to the back of the thyroid
- Adrenal glands, located above the kidneys
- Pancreas
- Carotid body, near the fork of the carotid artery in the neck

Procedures involving the endocrine system are covered by codes **60000** through **60699.**

Thyroidectomy

A thyroidectomy is the surgical removal of part or all of the thyroid gland for the purposes of treatment or removal of diseased tissue. A related procedure is the **thyroid lobectomy**, which involves the removal of one of the two lobes the thyroid gland is divided into and may also include the removal of the isthmus. When coding these types of procedures, there are a few important factors that must be considered. The first of these is the **amount of tissue** being removed. If only one lobe of the thyroid is removed, it is a **lobectomy**; if both lobes of the thyroid are being removed, either partially (**subtotal**) or completely (**total**), it is a thyroidectomy. Check which **additional procedures** are included, such as a contralateral subtotal lobectomy or dissection of the lymph nodes of the neck.

Nervous System

Anatomical Structures

The nervous system is the complex, interlinked system of tissues and organs that transmits and receives the signals that control all bodily functions, both conscious and unconscious. The nervous system is divided into two parts: the **central nervous system** and the **peripheral nervous system.**

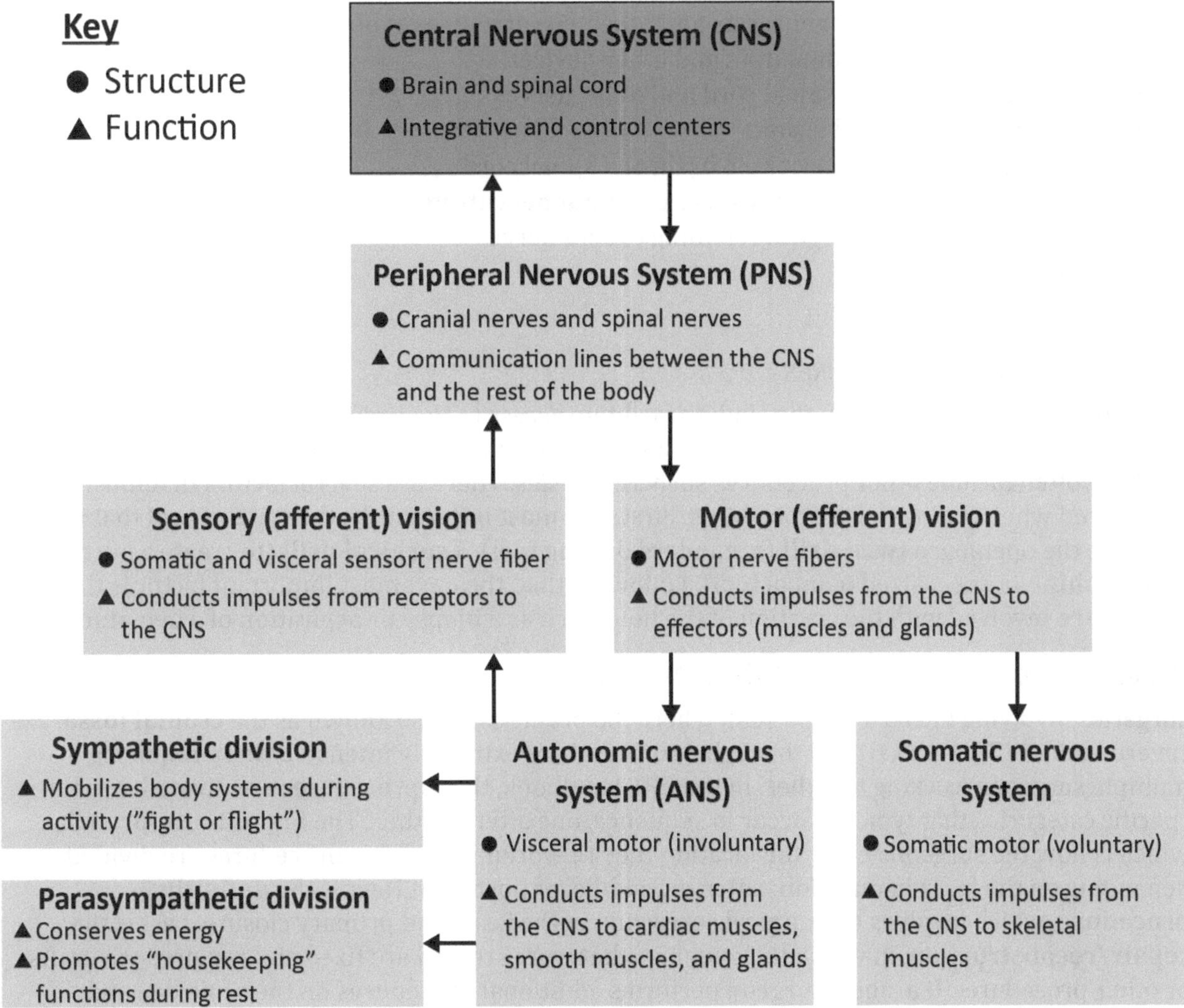

The central nervous system consists of the **brain,** the large mass of neural matter located inside the skull that controls the body; and the **spinal cord**, a long tubular structure that runs down along the vertebrae through the **spinal canal**, the open space behind the vertebral bodies. The central nervous system serves as the body's main control center and communication system. The peripheral nervous system is the term used for all of the other nerves that branch off of the spinal cord, which control the various muscles, organs, and other systems within the body.

Procedures

Procedures involving the nervous system and its associated structures are covered by CPT codes **61000** through **64999** in the CPT handbook, which are divided into related headings and subheadings throughout the section based on anatomical relevance. Procedures in this section include the following:

- Injection, drainage, and aspiration procedures on the skull, spine, and nerves
- Surgery of the skull, meninges, and brain
- Surgical treatment of aneurysms and other vascular disease of the brain
- Implanting of neurostimulators and other devices
- Decompression of the spinal cord and other nerves
- Excision of spinal cord lesions
- Stereotactic radiosurgery of the brain and spinal cord
- Chemical destruction of nerves (i.e., **chemodenervation**)
- **Neurorrhaphy**, the surgical rejoining of split nerves
- Nerve and vein grafts

Skull

Cranial Puncture Procedures

Holes are sometimes created in the skull to facilitate access to the tissues within or to treat issues inside the skull. The codes that cover these sorts of procedures are **61105** through **61253** in CPT, and they often include other procedures such as biopsies. There are several factors that must be considered when coding these procedures. First, and most importantly, the **type of tool** that is used to create the opening: a **twist drill** (a standard drilling tool), a **surgical drill** (to create a burr hole), or a **trephine** (a specialized manual tool). Following that, the next most important factor is the **procedure** involved with the creation of the hole, such as a biopsy or aspiration of a hematoma.

Surgical Procedures Involving Base of Skull

Surgeries involving the base of the skull where the brain rests, also known as the **cranial fossa**, are covered under CPT codes 61580 through 61619 and are extremely intensive, often requiring multiple surgeons working together. In the CPT handbook, these procedures are divided into three specific categories that typically occur in sequence, one after another. The first is the **approach**, which is how the surgeons enter the location they're working in. These procedures are divided depending on the fossa in question: anterior, middle, or posterior. Next is the **definitive procedure**, which involves the surgical correction of the issue and primary closure. Last is the **repair/reconstruction**, in which the openings that were created are fixed and repaired via grafts or other procedures. If a single surgeon performs additional procedures on the same day and during the same surgical session that are not a component of the primary procedure, modifier 51 may be appended to the minor code according to Medicare's National Corrective Coding Initiative (NCCI) edits.

Meninges

The brain and spinal cord do not rest directly against the bones protecting them. They are covered with a protective series of membranes referred to as the **meninges.** The meninges are made up of three layers: the **dura mater**, the outermost layer that rests against the bones of the skull and the vertebrae and contains the blood supply; the **arachnoid**, which is a thin connective layer that forms the boundary between the outer and inner layers of the meninges; and the **pia mater**, the thin and delicate membrane that attaches to the brain and spinal cord. The space between the pia mater and the arachnoid mater is referred to as the **subarachnoid space** and contains **cerebrospinal fluid (CSF)**, a colorless fluid that provides a cushioning effect.

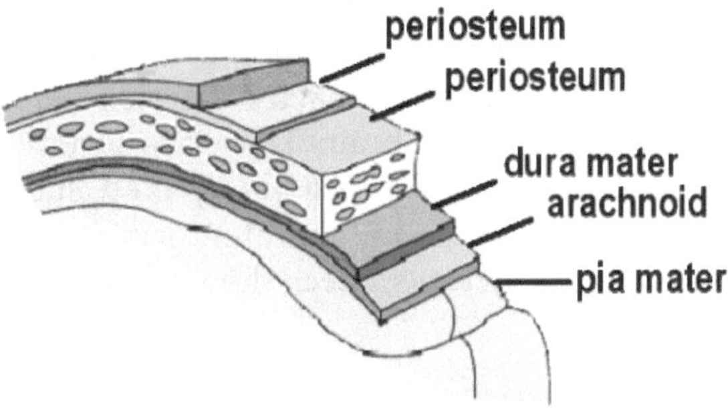

BRAIN

ANATOMY

The brain is a highly complex organ, located inside the skull, that serves as the central point of the nervous system, effectively functioning as a biological computer in control of all of the body's other organs and systems. In CPT, the brain is divided into two **hemispheres** (left and right) and consists of six regions:

- The **frontal lobes** (the large and frontmost part of the brain)
- The **parietal lobes** (the middle of the brain)
- The **temporal lobes** (located to the sides and below the parietal lobes)
- The **occipital lobes** (located toward the rear of the skull)
- The **cerebellum** (the mass located just below the occipital lobes)
- The **brain stem** (where the brain meets the spinal cord)

The brain also contains a variety of other structures and glands, such as the **hypothalamus**, **thalamus**, **pituitary gland**, **pons**, and **medulla**, that help to regulate the body's various hormonal systems.

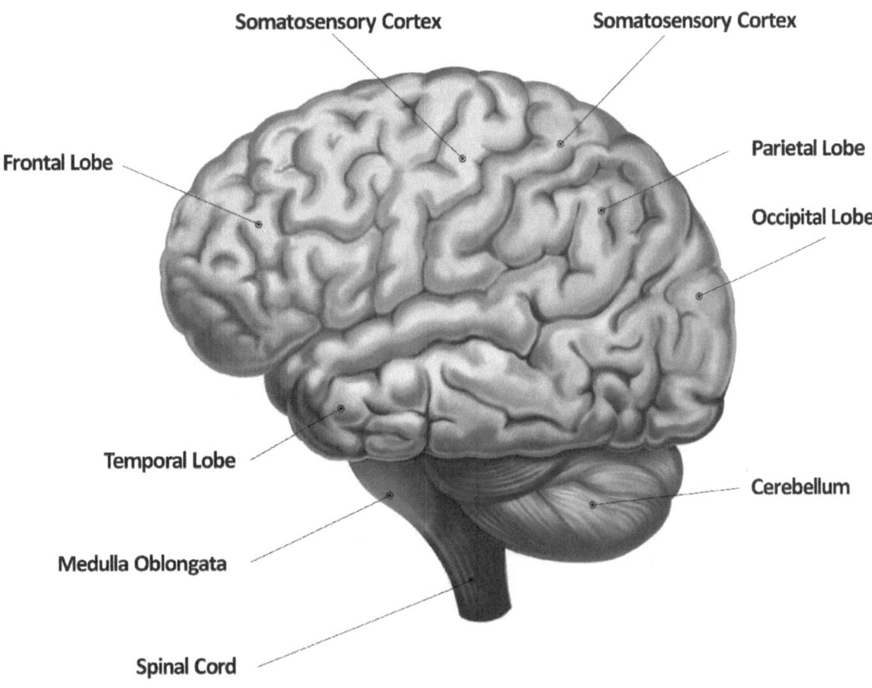

Surgical Treatment of Aneurysms and Related Conditions

Conditions involving the brain's blood vessels typically require surgical interventions, which in CPT are covered by codes **61680** through **61711**. These codes include surgery for aneurysms, carotid cavernous fistulas (an abnormal connection between the carotid artery and the cavernous sinus), and **arteriovenous malformation** (a tangle of connected arteries and veins), as well as vascular disease procedures on the skull, meninges, and brain. There are several factors to consider when coding these procedures. First, confirm the **condition being fixed**, such as a malformation or aneurysm. For malformations, check the **location** (supratentorial, infratentorial, or dural) and whether it's **simple** or **complex.** For aneurysms, check the **approach** (e.g., intracranial, cervical) to select the correct code.

Procedures Involving Cerebrospinal Fluid (CSF) Shunts

A CSF shunt is a medical implant that is placed inside the body to relieve pressure on the brain caused by an excess of CSF. Procedures involving CSF shunts typically involve either the placement of a new shunt, the replacement or revision (such as for an obstructed valve) of an existing shunt, or the complete removal of the system without replacement. In addition to those general categories, it is important to take several factors into account when coding these procedures. When a shunt is being placed, confirm the **location of the shunt** and the **method** with which it is placed. In addition, pay attention to the parenthetical notes under the replacement and revision and complete removal procedure codes.

Spine

Spinal Puncture Procedures

Spinal puncture procedures use a needle or similar tool that is inserted into the spinal canal for treatment purposes, typically involving injections, drainage, or aspiration. Injections into the spine typically involve injections into the **spinal epidural space**, which is a layer between the dura mater and the actual bony portion of the spine. These procedures are often referred to as **epidurals**, and they can involve the injection of contrast agents, therapeutic drugs, or anesthetics. Aspiration of the spine, or a **spinal tap**, is the removal of CSF or other material from the spine, whereas drainage involves removal of excess CSF.

When coding these procedures, note the key terms used by CPT in describing the procedure. These terms cover the **method** (percutaneous, endoscopic, and open) and **method of visualization** (either **indirect** via imaging guidance or **direct** via eyesight or endoscope).

Laminotomy and Laminectomy Procedures

Both laminotomy and laminectomy procedures involve the removal of the **lamina** (the vertebral arch that protects the spinal cord) of one or more vertebrae to reduce pressure on the spinal cord. The difference is the amount removed: Laminotomies are partial, whereas a laminectomy removes the entire arch. There are several factors involved in coding these procedures. First, check the **section of the spine**, such as cervical or lumbar, where the procedure is being performed. In addition, several codes are designed for only a single interspace. These codes will have add-on codes for additional interspaces that are covered by the procedure. For example, the laminotomy of three cervical interspaces would be reported using CPT codes 63020, +63035, +63035.

Spinal Cord

Excision of Intraspinal Lesions

An intraspinal lesion is a mass or tumor that is formed off the spinal cord or meninges and protrudes into the spinal canal. Treatment for intraspinal lesions is always surgical and may involve partial removal of the vertebral body. There are several factors that must be taken into consideration when selecting the proper codes for these procedures. First, check the **location of the lesion** that will be removed to determine whether it's **extradural** (outside the dura mater) or **intradural** (within the dura mater). Next, check the **location on the spine**: cervical, thoracic, lumbar, or sacral. Finally, check the **approach** that the surgeon or surgeons take to reach the lesion. CPT codes 63300 through 63307 are for a single segment, so if the surgery covers multiple segments, use the add-on code **63308** for each additional segment.

Stereotactic Radiosurgery of the Spine

Stereotactic radiosurgery is a type of specialized, nonsurgical radiation therapy used to inactivate or eradicate small tumors and other abnormalities within the brain and spinal cord, typically by applying precision doses of high-level radiation to the target. Codes in this section are used for the actual procedure. Treatment planning, dosimetry, and other treatment management by the oncologist can be found in codes **77261** through **77799**. These codes also include any planning, dosimetry, targeting, positioning, and blocking performed by the surgeon. It should be noted that the primary code, **63620**, should only be reported once per course of treatment, with the add-on code **63621** being reported once for each additional lesion, per course of treatment, and only up to a maximum of twice for the entire course of treatment, regardless of the number of lesions treated.

Extracranial, Peripheral, and Autonomic Nerves

Anatomical Purposes

This section of CPT covers three categories of nerves, each with their own part to play in the body: extracranial, peripheral, and autonomic nerves. Extracranial nerves are nerves that emerge from the skull, controlling and receiving signals to and from structures in the head, such as the eyes, ears, tongue, and nose. Peripheral nerves, meanwhile, are the nerves that branch off from the spinal cord and connect the central nervous system to the rest of the body, and they serve as sensors and to control the body's muscles (which are handled by **somatic nerves**) and organs. Finally, autonomic nerves are the parts of the peripheral nervous system that control the organs and glands involuntarily, allowing for the cardiovascular, respiratory, and digestive systems to operate without conscious input from the brain.

Procedures

Procedures specifically involving extracranial, peripheral, and autonomic nerves are covered by CPT codes **64400** through **64999,** which are divided into subheadings based on the specific type of procedure. Procedures in this section include the following:

- Introduction and injection procedures to anesthetize nerves (known as **nerve blocks**)
- Implantation, revision, and replacement of neurostimulators
- Destruction of nerves via chemical and other means, particularly **chemodenervation**
- Surgical exploration and decompression of nerves and nerve tissue
- Transection or avulsion of nerves
- **Neurorrhaphy**, the surgical rejoining of split nerves, including the use of grafts

Note that while this CPT code range contains the surgical destruction and exploration of nerves and nerve tissue, the destruction and exploration of the cranial nerve specifically can be reported with CPT codes 61458 and 61460.

Nerve Block

A nerve block is a procedure in which an anesthetic agent is injected into a nerve, nerve branch, or **nerve plexus** (a branching network of interlinked nerves) to block signals from a localized area for therapeutic or treatment purposes. There are several factors that must be accounted for when coding these procedures. First, check whether **imaging guidance** is required, because this will affect which type of code is used. Although most of the codes will have imaging guidance coded separately, some have it included in the procedure. Next, check **which nerve** is being injected. Finally, check **how many units or injections** are required by the code.

For further clarification, see the chart located in the "Introduction/Injection of Anesthetic Agent" subheading in this section of the CPT handbook.

Neuroplasty

Neuroplasty is a surgical procedure that is performed to relieve painful pressure on nerves, typically by removing scar tissue around the local area to free the nerve. A particularly common use of this is for the treatment of **carpal tunnel syndrome** (compression of the median nerve of the hand). Neuroplasty procedures can also include **neurolysis** (temporary artificial degeneration of nerve fibers), exploration, decompression, and transposition of nerve tissue. When coding these procedures, take note of the **anatomical location** of the nerve that is being treated, and also any **additional procedures**, such as neurolysis or transposition, that are being performed as part of the procedure.

Eye and Ear

EYE/OCULAR ADNEXA

ANATOMICAL STRUCTURES

The eyes are the organs responsible for the collection and transmission of visual information to the brain (i.e., sight). The eyes are located in the curved **orbital** sections of the skull and consist of two sections: the **anterior** and **posterior**. The anterior section includes the **cornea**, the transparent covering of the front of the eye; the **iris**, the thin, muscle-controlled opening that forms the pupil; and the **lens**, the transparent, biconvex structure that focuses and refracts light. The posterior portion of the eye includes the jelly-like **vitreous humor** that fills the eye itself; the **retina**, which converts light into nerve signals; and the optic nerve. The eye is covered by the **sclera,** a whitish membrane that helps to protect the internal structures.

This section also covers the **adnexa**, or accessory structures of the eyes, including the muscles, the eyelids, and the **conjunctiva** (mucous membranes) and **lacrimal system** (tear-producing systems) that help lubricate them.

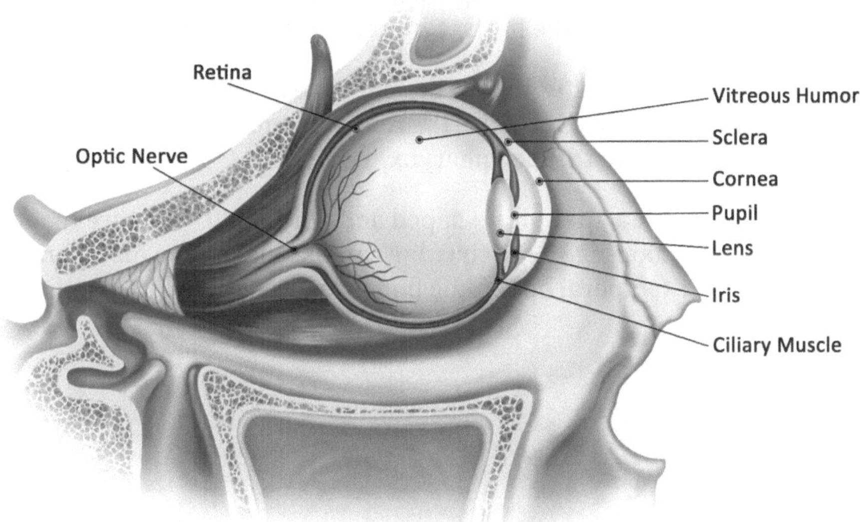

INTRAOCULAR LENS PROCEDURES

Intraocular lens procedures are procedures that involve the surgical removal and replacement of the lens, the part of the eye that focuses light on the retina. These procedures are typically performed to correct **cataracts**, a clouding and occlusion of the lens that typically occurs due to age or trauma. These procedures almost always include the insertion of a prosthetic lens to replace the damaged or diseased lens. There are several factors that must be accounted for when coding intraocular lens procedures. First, check whether the procedure is **extracapsular** or **intracapsular** (i.e., whether the tissue that covers the lens is to be left intact [extracapsular] or removed entirely [intracapsular]). Next, check if the procedure includes **stages**. Most of the procedures are done in a single stage, but code **66985** is a two-stage procedure in which the cataract is removed first, followed by the insertion of an intraocular lens prosthesis. In addition, take note of the parentheticals listed under some of the procedure descriptions for additional codes that may be needed to fully code the procedure.

Surgical Procedures Involving Extraocular Muscles

The extraocular muscles are a set of five muscles that are attached to the eye, keeping it in place and allowing it to move around in its orbit. Surgical procedures involving the extraocular muscles typically involve the correction of **strabismus**, a condition in which one or both eyes remain out of alignment. As with most surgical procedures, there are several factors that must be considered when selecting the proper codes. First, check **which muscle** the procedure is being performed on. If the procedure is performed on the horizontal or vertical muscles, check the **number of muscles** (one or two) that the procedure is performed on. In addition, check for **prior surgeries or conditions** in this area, such as a detached extraocular muscle or a previous eye surgery.

Auditory System

Anatomical Structures

The auditory system is the body system responsible for capturing and transmitting sound-based stimuli to the brain (i.e., hearing). The auditory system is located on the head and includes the ears and related anatomical structures. The **ear**, which is the main auditory organ, is divided into three sections, the **outer**, **middle**, and **inner ear**.

The outer ear is made up of the external cartilage and skin "funnel" of the **auricle**, the tube-like **external auditory canal** that leads to the fleshy **tympanic membrane**.

The tympanic membrane forms the outer wall of the middle ear, which is made up of the **tympanic cavity** that contains the three bones of the ear—the **malleus**, **incus**, and **stapes**—as well as the **eustachian tube**, which connects to the nasopharynx.

The inner ear contains the **cochlea**, the spiral-shaped and fluid-filled structure that connects to the auditory nerve; as well as the hoop-like **semicircular canals**, which help maintain balance. This area also includes parts of the temporal bones, the bones of the skull that the auditory system runs through.

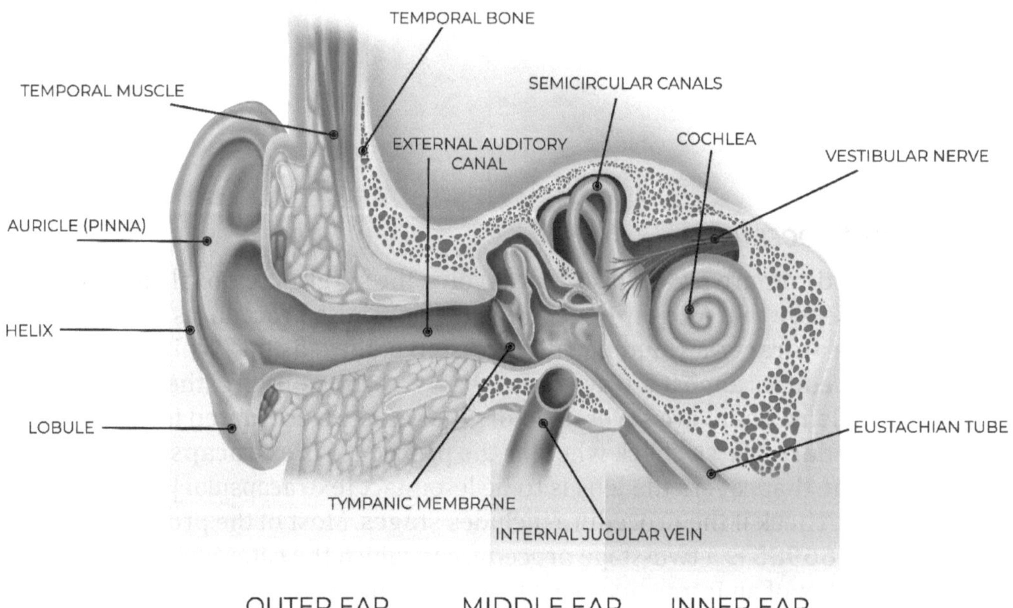

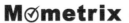

Tympanoplasty

A tympanoplasty is the surgical repair of a damaged or destroyed **tympanic membrane**. The tympanic membrane, commonly called the **eardrum**, is the fleshy covering located at the end of the external auditory canal that protects and transmits sound to the tympanic cavity. There are a few factors that must be considered when coding tympanoplasty procedures. First, check which **other procedures are or are not included** along with the tympanic membrane, such as a mastoidectomy or an antrotomy. In addition, check whether an **ossicular chain reconstruction** is or is not included in the procedure, because the associated codes are different from a standard tympanoplasty.

Operating Microscope

An operating microscope is a specialized type of microscope used by providers to visualize fine structures during a surgical procedure. This device is typically used for the purposes of conducting **microsurgery**, surgeries involving extremely small or delicate structures such as small nerves and tubes and parts of the ear, nose, and throat. Microsurgical techniques using an operating microscope are reported using code **69990**, which is an add-on code and cannot be reported individually. Do not report this code if magnifying loupes or corrected vision are used in the procedure. In addition, many codes from multiple sections include the use of an operating microscope in their procedure codes and thus do not require this code to be reported separately. See the description of code 69990 for a full list of codes that include microsurgery using an operating microscope.

Chapter Quiz

Ready to see how well you retained what you just read? Scan the QR code to go directly to the chapter quiz interface for this study guide. If you're using a computer, simply visit the bonus page at **mometrix.com/bonus948/cpc** and click the Chapter Quizzes link.

Evaluation and Management (E/M)

Transform passive reading into active learning! After immersing yourself in this chapter, put your comprehension to the test by taking a quiz. The insights you gained will stay with you longer this way. Scan the QR code to go directly to the chapter quiz interface for this study guide. If you're using a computer, simply visit the bonus page at **mometrix.com/bonus948/cpc** and click the Chapter Quizzes link.

New and Established Patients

Codes for office and outpatient services are often divided by whether the patient is **new** or **established**. According to CPT guidelines, the criteria for new and established patients are determined by the following:

- A **new** patient is a patient who has not received any professional services from the physician or qualified healthcare professional in question, nor from a physician or qualified healthcare professional in the same group practice with the exact same specialty and subspecialty, **within the past three years**.
- An **established** patient is a patient who has received professional services from the physician or qualified healthcare professional, or one in the same group practice with the exact same specialty and subspecialty, within the past three years. This includes advanced practice nurses or physician assistants working with the physician or healthcare professional.

Patient's History

A patient's history can be divided into three parts:

- The **history of present illness** (HPI) includes an evaluation of the patient's complaint, and—when applicable—includes the location, quality of discomfort, severity (often rated on a scale of 1-10), associated symptoms, how often the complaint occurs, when it began, and anything that makes it better or worse.
- A **review of systems** (ROS) allows the physician to select what other body systems are affected.
- The **past, family, and social history** (PFSH) evaluates a patient's past medical conditions, family health conditions, and tobacco and alcohol use.

When selecting an E/M code, be sure that the physician or other qualified healthcare professional is collecting a medically appropriate history from the patient based on their complaint.

Examination

Examinations are the physical or clinical inspection of a patient's affected areas or bodily systems. The body areas and organ systems are organized as followed: head (and face), neck, chest (and breasts and axillae), abdomen, genitalia (with the groin and buttocks), back, arms, legs, hands, feet, eyes, ears, nose, throat, mouth, cardiovascular system, respiratory system, gastrointestinal system, genitourinary system, musculoskeletal system, skin, neurological system, psychiatric, and hematological (and lymphatic and immunological). When selecting an E/M code, be sure that the physician or other qualified healthcare professional is collecting a medically appropriate examination from the patient based on their complaint.

Levels of Medical Decision-Making

According to the American Medical Association, medical decision-making (MDM) is a process in which the physician or other qualified healthcare professional establishes a diagnosis, evaluates the status of a condition, and/or selects a management option. The four levels of MDM are straightforward, low, moderate, and high. When considering which level of MDM a physician has performed, consider the following three elements:

- The number and complexity of problems that are addressed during the encounter.
- The amount and/or complexity of data to be reviewed and analyzed, including tests, medical records, and communication with an independent historian or healthcare professional.
- The risk of complications and/or morbidity or mortality of patient management associated with a diagnostic procedure or treatment, even when that procedure or treatment is not selected by the patient.

To determine the level of MDM, two of the three elements for that level of MDM must be met or exceeded.

Selection of Proper Categories for E/M Services

Effective January 1, 2023, code selection for outpatient, home health services, nursing facility care, inpatient, and observation services is either based on MDM with an appropriate history intake and examination, or based on time (with the exception of emergency services coding).

Medical Decision-Making

The level of MDM is based on 2 of 3 elements meeting or exceeding the requirements.

Element	Straightforward	Low
Problems addressed	Minimal • 1 self-limited or minor problem	Low • 2 or more self-limited or minor problems • 1 stable chronic illness • 1 acute, uncomplicated illness or injury • 1 stable acute illness • 1 acute, uncomplicated illness or injury requiring hospital inpatient or observation level of care
Data analyzed	Minimal or none	Limited (Must meet requirements of at least 1 out of 2 categories) **Category 1: Tests and documents** Any combination of 2 from the following: • Review of prior external note(s) from each unique source • Review of the result(s) of each unique test • Ordering of each unique test **Category 2: Assessment requiring independent historian**
Risks	Minimal risk of morbidity from additional diagnostic testing or treatment	Low risk of morbidity from additional diagnostic testing or treatment

Evaluation and Management (E/M)

Element	Moderate	High
Problems addressed	Moderate • 1 or more chronic illnesses with exacerbation, progression, or side effects from treatment • 2 or more stable, chronic illnesses • 1 undiagnosed new problem with uncertain prognosis • 1 acute illness with systemic symptoms • 1 acute, complicated injury	High • 1 or more chronic illnesses with severe exacerbation, progression, or side effects of treatment • 1 acute or chronic illness or injury that poses a threat to life or bodily function
Data analyzed	Moderate (Must meet requirements of at least 1 of 3 categories) **Category 1: Tests, documents, or independent historian(s)** Any combination of 3 from the following: • Review of prior external note(s) from each unique source • Review of the result(s) of each unique test • Ordering of each unique test • Assessment requiring an independent historian(s) **Category 2: Independent interpretation of tests** Independent interpretation of a test performed by another physician or other qualified health care professional (not separately reported). **Category 3: Discussion of management or test interpretation** Discussion with external physician or other qualified health care professional or appropriate source (not separately reported).	Extensive (Must meet the requirements of at least 2 out of 3 categories) **Category 1: Tests, documents, or independent historian(s)** Any combination of 3 from the following: • Review of prior external note(s) from each unique source • Review of the result(s) of each unique test • Ordering of each unique test • Assessment requiring an independent historian(s) **Category 2: Independent interpretation of tests** Independent interpretation of a test performed by another physician or other qualified health care professional (not separately reported). **Category 3: Discussion of management or test interpretation** Discussion with external physician or other qualified health care professional or appropriate source (not separately reported).
Risks	Moderate risk of morbidity from additional diagnostic testing or treatment	High risk of morbidity from additional diagnostic testing or treatment

Role of Time in E/M Procedures

According to the American Medical Association, when coding based on time, both face-to-face time spent with the patient, guardian, or family members and non-face-to-face time personally spent by the physician or other qualified healthcare provider on the day of the encounter should be accounted for when leveling an E/M service. For services 55 minutes or longer, use prolonged services code 99417 in conjunction with CPT codes 99205, 99215, 99245, 99345, 99350, and 99483. On the other hand, if in an outpatient setting, the time is spent supervising clinical staff who are evaluating the patients, only CPT code 99211 should be reported. Additionally, because a physician working in the emergency department may manage the care of multiple patients over an extended period, emergency services (CPT codes 99281 through 99285) cannot be reported based on time.

Place of Services

OFFICE AND OUTPATIENT SERVICES

Encounters for office and outpatient services are covered by codes **99202** through **99215** in CPT. Office and outpatient service codes are used to report E/M services in an office or outpatient facility. These services typically cover patients who visit a doctor's office or other outpatient facilities and who are **ambulatory** (able to move under their own power) or suffering from relatively minor conditions. These typically include face-to-face services rendered by physicians and other qualified health professionals. Patients are considered outpatients until they are admitted to a healthcare facility, such as a hospital or nursing facility. These codes do not include emergency care.

CODING OUTPATIENT PROCEDURES

Outpatient codes require a medically appropriate history and exam, and a leveled MDM or a documented note stating how much time was spent on the encounter to determine the proper E/M code. Refer to the following chart for a quick reference of the criteria for each code.

	Code	Decision-Making	Time (minimum)
New patient	99202	Straightforward	15 min
	99203	Low	30 min
	99204	Moderate	45 min
	99205	High	60 min
Established patient	99212	Straightforward	10 min
	99213	Low	20 min
	99214	Moderate	30 min
	99215	High	40 min

For new patient encounters lasting 75 minutes or longer, and for established patient encounters lasting 55 minutes or longer, use prolonged services code 99417 for each additional 15 minutes of total time. This code should always be used as an add-on code to CPT codes 99205 and 99215.

HOSPITAL OBSERVATION AND INPATIENT

OBSERVATION AND INPATIENT CARE PROCEDURES

A patient is designated as "observation status" in a hospital setting when the physician is unsure if the patient's condition requires further care by means of admission or can be safely discharged home. According to CMS guidelines, a patient may remain in observation status for a maximum of 48 hours. Inpatient care is when a patient is admitted into a hospital or similar medical facility for the purposes of treatment. Inpatient care may last for one or more days, and it may be preceded by a period of observation.

There are a few factors that may alter the use of inpatient care codes. If the patient is 28 days old or younger (a neonate), then use code 99477 instead of an inpatient code. If the initial inpatient encounter is performed by someone other than the admitting physician, refer to codes 99252 through 99255 for consultation codes, or 99231 through 99233 for subsequent hospital inpatient or observation care codes. If the patient is admitted and discharged on the same day, refer to codes 99234 through 99236.

Coding

Initial hospital inpatient or observation care codes require a medically appropriate history or examination, and a level of medical decision-making or documented total time to determine the proper codes. Refer to the following chart for a quick reference of the criteria for each code.

	Code	Decision-Making	Time (minimum)
Initial visit	99221	Straightforward or low	40 min
	99222	Moderate	55 min
	99223	High	75 min
Subsequent visits	99231	Straightforward or low	25 min
	99232	Moderate	35 min
	99233	High	50 min

For services 90 minutes or longer during initial hospital inpatient or observation care, and for services 65 minutes or longer during subsequent hospital inpatient or observation care, use prolonged services code 99418 for each additional 15 minutes of total time. This code should always be used as an add-on code to CPT codes 99223 and 99233.

Discharge Service Procedures

Discharge codes are used when a patient is cleared to leave the hospital after a period of observation and/or treatment. These codes include the final examination of a patient; discussion of the hospital stay; and preparation of any necessary referral forms, prescriptions, and discharge records. When coding, note the **amount of time** taken for the procedure because that determines which code is used. These codes are not to be used if the patient is admitted and discharged on the same day; if this occurs, see codes **99234** through **99236**. In addition, note the parentheticals underneath the code descriptions for additional contraindications and alternate codes.

Consults

A consult is a form of E/M service that involves another physician, specialist, or other appropriate medical provider being brought in to assist the initial provider. Consulting providers may recommend care or procedures for specific issues or take over in the place of the initial provider. A consult is only coded if it is initiated by a physician or other appropriate source, not by the patient or their family. Consults may be performed in office/outpatient and inpatient settings. Procedures performed during or after the initial consult should be reported separately using the appropriate procedure codes. If the procedure is mandated by a third party, use modifier **32** in addition to the consult procedure code.

Coding

Consultation codes, both office-based and inpatient, require either a medically appropriate history and/or examination, and a level of medical decision-making or documented total time to determine the proper codes. Refer to the following chart for a quick reference of the criteria for each code.

	Code	Decision-Making	Time (minimum)
Office-based	99242	Straightforward	20 min
	99243	Low	30 min
	99244	Moderate	40 min
	99245	High	55 min

	Code	Decision-Making	Time (minimum)
Inpatient	99252	Straightforward	35 min
	99253	Low	45 min
	99254	Moderate	60 min
	99255	High	80 min

For services 95 minutes or longer during inpatient or observation consultation, and for services 70 minutes or longer during an office or other outpatient consultation, use prolonged services code 99417 for each additional 15 minutes of total time. This code should always be used as an add-on code to CPT codes 99255 and 99245.

Emergency Department

Emergency department services are E/M services that are used when a patient is seen in the emergency department. CPT defines an emergency department as an organized, hospital-based facility for providing unscheduled episodic services, 24 hours a day, to patients requiring immediate medical care. Emergency department service codes also include a code for **directed emergency care** by ambulance or rescue personnel away from or en route to the hospital such as cardiac resuscitation, intubation of the airway, administration of intravenous fluids and injected drugs, and so on. Emergency department service codes do not cover services delivered during critical care.

Procedures and Coding

Emergency department codes require a medically appropriate history or examination and a level of medical decision-making to determine the proper codes. Refer to the following chart for a quick reference of the criteria for each code.

Code	Decision-Making
99282	Straightforward
99283	Low
99284	Moderate
99285	High

Unlike with other codes, total time spent and whether the patient is new or established are not considered when determining the level of service.

Critical Care

Critical care services are a type of E/M service used for direct delivery of medical care for a critically ill or injured patient by a qualified healthcare professional, often involving high-complexity decision-making to assess and treat life-threatening deterioration or damage. This also covers transport of critically ill or injured patients to or from a hospital or other facility. The following services are included in critical care: interpreting cardiac output measurements, chest x-rays, pulse oximetry, blood gases, collection and interpretation of physiological data, temporary transcutaneous pacing, ventilatory management, and vascular access procedures. Critical care services rendered to infants 29 days (about 4 weeks) through 71 months (about 6 years) of age are reported with pediatric critical care codes 99471 through 99476. Critical care services rendered to neonates 28 days of age or younger are reported with neonate critical care codes 99468 and 99469.

Coding

When coding critical care services, the key factor to consider is **time**; the primary code (**99291**) is for the first 30 to 74 minutes of service, whereas the add-on code **99292** is used for each additional

30-minute block. When coding these procedures, translate the given time into minutes and round up each 30-minute block. For example, a critical care service that lasts for 1 hour and 45 minutes would translate into 105 minutes, resulting in 99291 once and 99292 twice (74 + 30 + 1, which rounds up to 30).

Common procedures performed during critical care services that are reported separately include CPR (**92950**), intubation (**31500**), and central line placement (**36620** through 36640, 36555, 36556, and 36560).

Nursing Facilities

Nursing facility services are E/M procedures used for patients in long-term care facilities, intermediate care facilities, and other convalescent or rehabilitative facilities. These facilities provide around-the-clock care for resident patients, often including a multidisciplinary plan of care. This also includes facilities that provide medical psychotherapy and similar treatments. These codes only cover medical care at the facility. For codes focused on care plan oversight for facility residents, see codes **99379** and **99380.** If a patient is admitted to a nursing facility in the process of an encounter at another site, such as a hospital, all the E/M services provided in conjunction with that admission are considered part of the initial nursing facility care if they are performed on the same date. If a patient is discharged from inpatient status on the same date as admission or readmission to a nursing facility, use hospital inpatient discharge day management codes **99238** or **99239** as appropriate.

Procedures and Coding

Nursing facility care codes require a medically appropriate history or examination and a level of medical decision-making to determine the proper codes. When using total time on the date of the encounter, the time listed for each code must be met or exceeded. Refer to the following chart for a quick reference of the criteria for each code.

	Code	Decision-Making	Time
Initial visit	99304	Low	25 min
	99305	Moderate	35 min
	99306	High	45 min
Subsequent visits	99307	Straightforward	10 min
	99308	Low	15 min
	99309	Moderate	30 min
	99310	High	45 min

For services 60 minutes or longer, use prolonged services code 99418 in conjunction with CPT codes 99306 and 99310 for each additional 15 minutes of total time.

Home and Residence Services

Home or residence visits, including domiciliary, rest home (e.g., boarding home), or custodial care services, are used to report evaluation and management services provided in a private residence or short-term accommodation, such as an assisted-living facility, treatment facility, or group home. It should be noted that the procedures coded in this section of CPT only cover E/M inside the facility. These codes only cover the E/M services provided, not the facility's actual services. For codes focused on care plan oversight for home health agencies, see codes **99374** and **99375.** For hospice agencies, see codes **99377** and **99378.**

PROCEDURES AND CODING

Home and residence service codes require a medically appropriate history or examination, and a level of medical decision-making to determine the proper codes. When using total time on the date of the encounter, the time listed for each code must be met or exceeded. Additionally, any travel time should not be considered when selecting a code level based on time. Refer to the following chart for a quick reference of the criteria for each code.

	Code	Decision-Making	Time
New patient	99341	Straightforward	15 min
	99342	Low	30 min
	99344	Moderate	60 min
	99345	High	75 min
Established patient	99347	Straightforward	20 min
	99348	Low	30 min
	99349	Moderate	40 min
	99350	High	60 min

For services 90 minutes or longer for a new patient or 75 minutes or longer for an established patient, use prolonged services code 99417 in conjunction with CPT codes 99345 and 99350 for each additional 15 minutes of total time.

PREVENTATIVE MEDICINE

Preventative medicine is a periodic evaluation of infants, children, adolescents, and adults, and is commonly referred to as an annual physical or well-woman exam. These services are meant to evaluate the overall health and well-being of the patient, identify any potential health problems before they fully manifest, provide counseling and risk factor reduction interventions based on PFSH (past, family, and social history), and the ordering of laboratory/diagnostic procedures and tests. Although immunizations, laboratory tests, and screenings are commonly performed in conjunction with a preventative service, these procedures are reported separately from the evaluation and management code.

PROCEDURES AND CODING

When selecting a preventative medicine E/M, first identify whether the patient is new or established, because this is how the categories are initially divided. Second, check the **age** of the patient; procedure codes in this category are divided by patient age. These codes include counseling, anticipatory guidance, and risk reduction interventions provided during the procedure. If an abnormality or pre-existing medical condition is encountered during the evaluation but is not significant enough to require additional work or require a problem-oriented E/M service, it should not be reported.

Non-Face-to-Face Services

Types

Non-face-to-face E/M services involve providers monitoring or reviewing patient status via long-distance methods, often without seeing patients directly. E/M services in this category include the following:

- **Telephone services**, in which qualified healthcare providers speak with patients or receive information over the phone
- **Online digital services**, which are patient-initiated services with a physician or qualified health provider over electronic communication such as secure email or electronic health records
- **Interprofessional consultations**, a type of consultation performed via telephone, internet-based, or electronic health record services
- **Digitally stored data services** and **remote physiological monitoring**, in which remote devices (such as those in the patient's home) are interrogated for physiological data
- **Remote physiologic monitoring treatment management services**, in which the results from a remote monitoring device are used to manage a patient's treatment plan.

The devices used for these codes must be cleared by the Food and Drug Administration (FDA) before use, and all medical information transmitted must comply with HIPAA requirements.

Coding

Although non-face-to-face services encompass a wide variety of procedures and methodologies, many of them share similar factors that influence the selection of proper codes. A major component of these services, after the type of service is determined, is **time**. Each type of non-face-to-face E/M service, except digitally stored data services and remote physiological monitoring, requires a recorded amount of time in minutes, each having different ranges of time for each specific code. For digitally stored data services and remote physiological monitoring, code selection is based on the type of data being collected, the duration of monitored time, initial set-up of equipment, or patient education.

Neonatal and Pediatric Care

Newborn Care Services

Newborn care services are E/M codes used for dealing with newborn children, which are defined by CPT as an age range from birth through the first 28 days. These codes include services such as maternal and fetal history, physical examinations of the newborn, ordering of diagnostic tests and treatments, family meetings, and documentation. These codes cover care, not procedures performed on newborns (such as circumcision). Those codes are reported separately to the care service codes. If a newborn patient is later admitted for intensive care or additional critical care on the same day that one of these codes is used, report the appropriate E/M code for the admission with modifier 25 alongside the newborn service code.

Delivery/Birthing Room Attendance and Resuscitation Services

The "Newborn Care Services" section also includes delivery/birthing room attendance and resuscitation services, in which a doctor or other qualified health professional is in attendance and present at the birth to provide the initial stabilization of the newborn. This code, **99464**, may be reported in conjunction with 99221, 99222, 99291, 99460, 99468, and 99477.

This section also includes the code if the aforementioned health professional is required to perform CPR on a newborn postdelivery in the event of inadequate cardiac or respiratory output. Other procedures for resuscitation, such as intubation, are reported separately. This code, **99465**, is not reported in conjunction with 99464; it supersedes that one when it is used.

Intensive Care

Coding Inpatient Neonatal Intensive Care Services and Pediatric and Neonatal Critical Care Services

Inpatient neonatal and pediatric and neonatal critical care service codes are used when a critically ill **neonate** (a child aged 28 days or younger) or a **pediatric** (a child aged 29 days through 5 years of age) patient is put into the pediatric intensive care unit or the neonatal intensive care unit. The codes in this section are divided by age: 28 days or younger, 29 days to 24 months, and 2 to 5 years old. A variety of codes are included in this section, including the following: vascular access procedures, airway and ventilation management, monitoring/interpretation of blood gases and oxygen saturation, car seat evaluation, transfusion of blood components, oral or nasogastric tube placement, suprapubic bladder aspiration, bladder catheterization, and lumbar puncture. All other services should be reported separately.

Coding Continuing Intensive Care Services for Neonates

The use of initial and continuing intensive care service E/M codes is intended for neonates and infants who are not critically ill but still require intensive observation, intervention, and continuing care. These are typically used for premature newborns or newborn children with a low birth weight. These services include vital sign monitoring, heat maintenance, nutritional adjustments, and observation by a healthcare team directed by a physician. Procedures listed for neonatal and pediatric critical care codes are also bundled with these codes, and they should not be reported separately. These codes are reported once per day, unless the neonate or infant's condition improves to the point that intensive care is no longer required.

Prolonged Services

Prolonged services are E/M procedures in which a physician or other qualified healthcare provider performs prolonged or extended service or services beyond what is typically required in an inpatient or outpatient setting. Such services are reported in addition to the primary procedure and cover procedures that are performed with direct patient contact, without direct patient contact, or involving clinical staff or other qualified healthcare professional supervision. These codes only apply to E/M services or psychotherapy services; other services that are provided are not counted toward the prolonged services. Any medications or supplies used or additional procedures performed during the prolonged services should be coded alongside the prolonged services codes.

Coding

When reporting prolonged total time, utilize CPT codes 99417 and 99418. CPT code 99417 is reported for outpatient services, office consultations, or other outpatient evaluation and management services. On the other hand, CPT code 99418 is reported for an inpatient evaluation and management service. Report these codes to indicate that the highest level of service has been exceeded by at least 15 minutes. For example, if a patient is evaluated at an urgent care facility and the physician documents a total time of 105 minutes, report CPT codes 99205, 99417 × 3. Because prolonged service codes are add-on codes, they should never be reported on their own.

Care Management Evaluation and Management Services

Care management E/M services are rendered to patients with a single high-risk disease or multiple chronic conditions residing at home or in a domiciliary, rest home, or assisted-living facility. This includes establishing, implementing, revising, or monitoring the care plan, coordinating the care of other professionals and agencies, and educating the patient about their condition, care plan, or prognosis. Within the care management E/M services section of CPT are three subcategories: Principal Care Management Services, Complex Chronic Care Evaluation and Management Services, and Chronic Care Evaluation and Management Services. Chronic conditions may be continuous or episodic but are expected to last at least 12 months or until the death of the patient. In addition, the condition or conditions should place the patient at significant risk of exacerbation, decline, or death. **Complex** care management refers to chronic issues requiring multiple specialties and those that limit daily activities, complicate care, or require social support.

Coding

Coding principal care management services requires the following:

- One complex chronic condition that is expected to last at least 3 months, and that places the patient at significant risk of hospitalization, acute exacerbation/decompensation, functional decline, or death. The condition requires development, monitoring, or revision of a disease-specific care plan.
- The condition requires frequent adjustments in the medication regimen, or the management of the condition is unusually complex due to comorbidities.
- There is ongoing communication and care coordination between relevant practitioners furnishing care.

Coding chronic care and complex chronic care procedures requires the following:

- There are multiple chronic conditions that last for 12 months or until the death of the patient.
- The conditions place the patient at a significant risk of death, acute exacerbation, or decline.
- A comprehensive care plan is established, implemented, revised, or monitored, which includes specific and achievable goals for each condition that are measurable and relevant to the patient's lifestyle.

Complex care management has two additional criteria:

- Moderate- or high-complexity medical decision-making
- 60 minutes of clinical staff time per calendar month directed by a qualified healthcare professional or performed by a physician

Both categories are coded based on the **amount of time** of the encounter. Complex services have much longer time allotments, and the add-on code **99489** should be used for every 30-minute block after the initial 60 minutes. For example, a complex care service that lasts for 99 minutes uses codes 99487 and 99489 once (60 + 39, rounded down to 30).

Transitional Care

Transitional care services are E/M procedures involving the transition of a patient with medical or psychosocial problems from an inpatient hospital setting (acute or long term), partial hospital setting, observation, or skilled nursing facility to a community setting (such as the patient's home, a rest home, or an assisted-living facility). These patients must have medical conditions that require a moderate to high level of medical decision-making (as defined by CPT). These services include at least one face-to-face visit within the specified timeframe, any additional non-face-to-face services performed by the physician or qualified healthcare professional and/or clinical staff, and coordination of care between multiple disciplines.

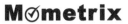

Coding

In order for transitional care procedures to be eligible for coding, they must include certain elements. These include the following, as laid out by CPT guidelines:

- Communication in the form of direct, electronic, or telephone contact between the patient or patient's caregiver within 2 business days of discharge
- Medical decision-making of moderate (for code **99495**) or high (for code **99496**) complexity within the service period
- A face-to-face visit within 7 (for code **99496**) or 14 (for code **99495**) calendar days after the date of discharge

Procedures of this type involving high complexity only use code **99496** for the face-to-face visit within 7 days. All other instances of transitional care that involve face-to-face visits within 8 to 14 days use code **99495**, regardless of the complexity of medical decision-making.

Case Management

Case management services are the E/M procedures that are used when a physician or other qualified healthcare professional is directly caring for and initiating, coordinating, managing, or supervising additional healthcare services needed by the patient. This often involves conferences, either face-to-face or indirectly, between the physician, their team of healthcare professionals, and the patient and their family. When coding these procedures, the codes separate nonphysician qualified healthcare professionals from physicians: If a face-to-face conference with the patient is performed by the overseeing physician, that physician reports using the appropriate E/M procedure code.

Care Plan Oversight

Care plan oversight services are E/M procedures that cover recurrent supervision of a patient by a physician or other skilled healthcare provider. These codes are used for the supervision of multidisciplinary care in home healthcare environments, hospices, or nursing facilities. Such services include review of care plans and laboratory reports; communication with healthcare professionals, family members, legal guardians, and caregivers; modification or adjustment of medical treatment plans; and adjustment of medical therapy. These codes are divided by location of the patient and the time involved in the actual act of supervision. Care plan oversight of assisted-living facilities or hospice agencies uses codes separate from these.

Chapter Quiz

Ready to see how well you retained what you just read? Scan the QR code to go directly to the chapter quiz interface for this study guide. If you're using a computer, simply visit the bonus page at **mometrix.com/bonus948/cpc** and click the Chapter Quizzes link.

Anesthesia

Transform passive reading into active learning! After immersing yourself in this chapter, put your comprehension to the test by taking a quiz. The insights you gained will stay with you longer this way. Scan the QR code to go directly to the chapter quiz interface for this study guide. If you're using a computer, simply visit the bonus page at **mometrix.com/bonus948/cpc** and click the Chapter Quizzes link.

Time Reporting

Anesthesia time refers to the amount of time that an individual is placed under anesthesia for a procedure in the operating room or an equivalent area. During this time, the patient is under the care of the **anesthesiologist**, a medical professional specially trained in the administration of anesthetics. Procedures involving anesthesia will have an amount of time listed, either in whole or in part, as part of the procedure notes. As outlined by CPT, anesthesia time begins with the time it takes the anesthesiologist to prepare the patient for the induction of anesthesia while in the operating room or procedure room, and it ends when the anesthesiologist is officially no longer in personal attendance.

Procedures Included or Coded Separately from Anesthesia Procedures

Anesthesia procedure codes include a variety of additional services that will likely be used during the administration and monitoring of an anesthetized patient. These services are performed under the supervision of the physician in charge, and they vary widely. These include the use of supplementation of local anesthesia; preoperative and postoperative visits; anesthesia care during the actual procedure; the administration of fluid and/or blood; as well as forms of monitoring such as temperature, blood pressure, oximetry, electrocardiogram, capnography, and others. Some unusual forms of monitoring may also be used, including intra-arterial catheters (**36245 through 36248**), central venous catheters (**36555 through 36573**), Swan-Ganz catheters (**93503**), and endotracheal intubation (**31500**). These unusual services are coded separately.

Qualifying Circumstances

Qualifying circumstance codes are used when anesthesia must be administered under extreme or otherwise difficult circumstances based on the condition of the patient or the circumstances of the operation. These may include extreme age (young or old); the requirement of **full-body hypothermia** (cooling the body down to a very low temperature); the use of **controlled hypotension** (artificially lowering blood pressure); or conditions that would mean significant threat to the patient's life, health, or body parts if there's a delay. Qualifying circumstance codes are all add-on codes, meaning they are used in conjunction with anesthesia codes and cannot be coded on their own.

General and Monitored Anesthesia Care

Anesthesia is typically divided into two different categories based on the intended outcome. For **general anesthesia**, a patient is placed into a sleep-like state of unconsciousness for the duration of the operation and is brought out of it during recovery. **Conscious sedation**, also known as **moderate sedation** or **monitored anesthesia care (MAC)**, is a form of anesthesia in which the patient remains conscious enough to follow instructions but is generally calm and unable to feel pain. When coding anesthesia procedures that use the phrase "requires anesthesia," assume that the procedure is using MAC unless general anesthesia is explicitly mentioned.

Physical Status Modifiers

Physical status modifiers are modifiers, appended after an anesthesia code, that indicate the general level of health or status of the patient undergoing anesthesia. These modifiers are listed as P1 through P6 and are mandatory unless the billing is performed through Medicare. The modifiers are consistent with the guidelines established by the American Society of Anesthesiologists for ranking physical status, and they are as follows:

- **P1:** A healthy patient
- **P2:** A patient with a mild systemic disease
- **P3:** A patient with a severe systemic disease
- **P4:** The same as P3, but the disease is a constant threat to life
- **P5:** A patient that is not expected to survive without the operation
- **P6:** A declared brain-dead patient whose organs are being removed for donation

Common CPT Modifiers Used for Anesthesia Codes

Anesthesia procedure codes may require additional modifiers depending on the circumstances surrounding the procedure. These modifiers are appended to the end of a procedure code when applicable and are typically used for MAC during a surgical procedure. These codes are not always required for every procedure; they are required for atypical circumstances, such as when a procedure must end before completion or if unusual methods must be used. Common CPT modifiers include the following:

- **23:** Unusual anesthesia
- **47:** Anesthesia performed by surgeon
- **53:** Discontinued procedure (in this case, meaning the anesthesia itself is discontinued)
- **59:** Distinct procedural service
- **73:** Discontinued outpatient procedure prior to anesthesia administration
- **74:** Discontinued outpatient procedure subsequent to anesthesia administration

HCPCS Level II Modifiers

These modifiers, found in the HCPCS book, are some of the most commonly used modifiers for anesthesia procedures. These alphabetical and alphanumeric codes are typically used for MAC during a surgical procedure, and they help to properly describe the procedure as presented. Several of these codes are used when one or more certified registered nurse anesthetists (CRNAs) are involved in the procedure. These codes include the following:

- **AA**: Anesthesia performed personally by an anesthesiologist
- **AD:** Medical supervision by a physician of more than four concurrent anesthesia procedures
- **G8:** MAC for deep, complex, or highly invasive procedures
- **G9**: MAC for severe cardiopulmonary condition
- **QK**: Medical direction of two to four concurrent anesthesia procedures
- **QS**: MAC service
- **QX:** CRNA service with medical direction by an anesthesiologist
- **QY**: One CRNA service directed by an anesthesiologist
- **QZ**: CRNA service without direction by a physician

Anesthesia for Services

Anesthesia Codes for Surgical Procedures

The majority of codes in CPT's "Anesthesia" section cover procedures involving anesthesia for various types of surgical procedures. Codes in the "Anesthesia" section are divided primarily by anatomical location. It should be noted that, unless the anesthetic procedure code includes an actual description of a specific type of procedure (e.g., "Anesthesia for all closed procedures on lower leg, ankle, or foot"), the code description will typically include the phrase "**Not otherwise specified**," meaning that it covers a broad category of procedures. These codes will often have additional codes listed underneath to help indicate a more specific code, such as "Repair of ruptured Achilles tendon, with or without graft." When possible, select the most precise code for the procedure given.

Anesthesia Codes for Diagnostic Procedures

Several codes in CPT's "Anesthesia" section cover anesthesia for various types of diagnostic procedures. As with surgical codes, many of these procedures are grouped by anatomical location. When selecting codes for a diagnostic procedure, check the code description and give the procedure description for the proper terms used. Diagnostic procedures will include terms such as:

- Diagnostic
- Biopsy (such as percutaneous liver biopsy)
- Screening (such as screening colonoscopy)
- Procedures that end with the suffixes "-scopy" or "-graphy," such as arthroscopy or cholangiopancreatography

As noted in the "Surgery" sections of CPT, most surgical procedures will have a diagnostic portion included in their procedure code. This should be kept in mind when coding anesthesia for diagnostic procedures: Only code using anesthesia for a diagnostic procedure when a separate diagnostic procedure is being performed.

Anesthesia Codes for Radiological Procedures

Certain radiological procedures may require the use of anesthesia depending on the patient's health or condition. Radiological procedures mentioned in the "Anesthesia" section of CPT include the following:

- Diagnostic arteriography and venography
- Cardiac catheterization
- Radiation therapy
- Therapeutic intervention in the arterial, venous, or lymphatic systems
- Percutaneous, image-guided procedures on the spine and spinal cord

Note the specific anatomical area that the radiological procedure is being performed on, because that will influence which anesthesia code is selected for the procedure if required. These codes may or may not be included in the procedure code for the radiological procedure in question; read through the procedure code description before adding more codes.

Anesthesia Codes for Obstetric Procedures

Certain obstetric procedures may require the use of anesthesia depending on the procedure or the patient's health status. Many of the codes involved in this section of anesthesia will cover anesthesia involved in delivery, including the following:

- Vaginal delivery
- Cesarean delivery
- Hysterectomy, either following delivery or without labor
- Incomplete, missed, or induced abortions
- Neuraxial labor anesthesia, typically through an epidural catheter, during or in preparation for labor

Some of these codes (**01968** and **01969**) are add-on codes used in conjunction with earlier codes in this section. When coding these anesthesia procedures, confirm the primary procedure that is associated with the anesthesia code.

Chapter Quiz

Ready to see how well you retained what you just read? Scan the QR code to go directly to the chapter quiz interface for this study guide. If you're using a computer, simply visit the bonus page at **mometrix.com/bonus948/cpc** and click the Chapter Quizzes link.

Radiology

Transform passive reading into active learning! After immersing yourself in this chapter, put your comprehension to the test by taking a quiz. The insights you gained will stay with you longer this way. Scan the QR code to go directly to the chapter quiz interface for this study guide. If you're using a computer, simply visit the bonus page at **mometrix.com/bonus948/cpc** and click the Chapter Quizzes link.

Radiological Procedures

Radiological procedures are procedures that involve the use of various imaging techniques to diagnose and treat illnesses, often by using some form of directed energy. Radiological procedures cover a variety of methodologies that are used to observe internal body structure, including **ultrasound**, which uses high-frequency sound waves; **x-rays**, which use x-ray radiation; and **magnetic resonance imaging**, or **MRI**, which uses magnetic fields and radio waves. This section also includes **nuclear medicine**, which is when carefully measured traces of radioactive substances are used to locate, diagnose, and treat diseases. These procedures can be performed either separately as individual services, or in tandem with other procedures for the purposes of visualization or treatment.

Procedures in "Radiology" Section of CPT

Radiological procedures are covered by codes **70010** through **79999** in the CPT book, which are divided into related headings and subheadings throughout the section. Procedures in this section include the following:

Diagnostic radiology	Examination of body structures via radiological methods such as x-ray or MRI
Diagnostic ultrasound	Examination of various body structures via high-frequency sound waves
Radiological guidance	Radiological methods are used in conjunction with other procedures to guide treatment
Mammography	Radiological inspection of the mammary glands
Bone and joint studies	Includes bone densitometry and joint radiography
Radiation oncology	High-dose radiation of various sources used to treat cancer
Nuclear medicine	Radioactive substances introduced to the body to locate and diagnose disease

Diagnostic Radiology

Contrast Materials

Many diagnostic radiology procedures include a specifier: **without contrast material** or **with contrast material.** A contrast material is a substance, often injected, consumed, or otherwise introduced into the body, that has a different opacity from the surrounding soft tissue when viewed radiologically. When a procedure uses contrast material in a radiological procedure, introduced via injection into a vein, a joint, or the spinal canal, it uses a different CPT code. It should be noted, however, that if a contrast material is only administered orally (via the mouth) or rectally (via the rectum), then the procedure is technically considered "without contrast" for the purposes of coding the procedure.

Vascular Diagnostic Procedures

Vascular diagnostic procedures are when a contrast material is injected into a major artery, vein, or lymphatic vessel to properly view them to diagnose issues. These procedure codes are not to be used with interventional procedures because they are meant for diagnostic purposes alone, and intervention codes already bundle these services in. There are several factors to consider when coding these types of procedures. In addition to defining the **type of vessel being viewed** (such as an artery or vein), one must consider the **area being viewed**, such as an extremity. It is also important to check the **laterality** of the exam (i.e., whether it is unilateral or bilateral).

Diagnostic Ultrasound

Procedures and Coding

Diagnostic ultrasounds are radiological procedures that use ultra-high-frequency sound waves emitted and recorded by specialized machines to visualize a body's internal structures to examine and diagnose issues. These procedures cover a variety of soft tissues, including the circulatory system. When these procedures are coded, they may include several different scans, including an **A-mode** scan, a simple measurement of an echo to determine depth; a **B-mode** scan, a static two-dimensional image generated by sound; an **M-mode** scan, a recorded two-dimensional image in motion; or a real-time two-dimensional scan with motion.

Obstetric Ultrasound Procedures

Ultrasound imaging is commonly used for obstetric purposes, typically to visualize and document the fetus or fetuses for evaluation during gestation. Most codes involving these include real-time image documentation. There are several factors that must be considered when coding these procedures. First, check the **approach** used for the procedure, whether it's transabdominal or transvaginal. Next, check what else is **documented** during the procedure, such as an examination of the fetus's anatomy or the maternal structures. In addition, check for any **additional factors** that would affect the code selection, such as the trimester or number of fetuses. Finally, if the procedure is not an ultrasound, check what other factors are involved before selecting a final code.

Radiological Guidance Procedures

Radiological guidance procedures are those in which a radiological method—such as **fluoroscopy** (a type of x-ray that captures real-time movement of internal structures), **computed tomography** (a computerized x-ray that captures cross-sectional images of the body and its organs), or MRI—is used to help guide surgical or other treatments such as biopsies or tissue ablation. These procedures are divided by method of visualization. They are often accompanied by a list of codes that are either to be used in conjunction with or to avoid being reported with. When coding these procedures, it's extremely important to **check the parentheticals** to see whether the procedure code is reported separately from the procedure it provides guidance for. Several codes in the "Surgery" sections of CPT have these codes bundled in with the procedure.

Mammography

Mammograms are a specific type of radiological procedure that involves scanning the breasts for masses or lesions within the soft tissue. These procedures often involve a specialized scanning device that helps flatten the mass of the breast to improve the quality of the image. There are several factors that must be accounted for when coding these procedures. First, check the **specific procedure** being performed, such as a digital breast tomosynthesis or a mammogram. If the procedure is a mammogram, check whether the procedure is **diagnostic** or **screening**. Screening mammography is a routine procedure, whereas diagnostic mammography is used when a problem is suspected. Furthermore, check the **laterality** of the procedure (i.e., whether it is unilateral or bilateral).

Bone and Joint Studies

Radiological procedures involving the study of bones and joints are typically performed to study the density or shape of the bones or joints being scanned or to assess fractures, particularly of the vertebrae. There are a few factors that must be considered when coding these procedures. First, determine the **procedure** being performed. Next, check which **parts of the skeleton** are being scanned, if applicable. Certain procedures may call for a **dual-energy x-ray absorptiometry** scan, a type of bone density imaging that uses two x-ray beams of differing energy levels. For these procedures, only report a single procedure code, no matter how many sites are scanned.

Radiation Oncology

Radiation oncology is a set of radiological procedures that use carefully controlled high-intensity radiation from various sources to carefully treat or eliminate diseased or cancerous tissue in the body. Like other therapeutic treatments, radiation oncology procedure codes include related services such as the initial consultation, simulation of the procedure, dosimetry, clinical treatment management, and planning procedures and other special services, as well as normal follow-up care during treatment and in the three months after the completion of treatment. These codes do not cover preliminary consultation, the evaluation of the patient, or additional care provided by the radiologist, because those events use different codes from different sections of CPT.

Treatment Planning

Radiation treatment planning procedures cover the services involved in setting up a radiation treatment, such as interpretation of tests; determination of treatment time, dosage, and volume; and choice of modality. These codes are labeled as simple, intermediate, or complex in the procedural description to define the planning and simulation used in the procedure. **Simple** refers to a single treatment area, either for planning or simulation; **intermediate** refers to two separate treatment areas, often requiring three or more ports or multiple blocks; and **complex** involves three or more separate treatment areas, often including very complex blocking, compensation, or specialized treatment modality.

Radiation Treatment Delivery

Radiation treatment delivery procedures cover the actual administration of radiation during radiation oncology. These methods include x-rays, intensity-modulated radiation therapy (IMRT), electron beams, neutron beams, and proton beams. Similar to planning procedures, delivery procedures are labeled as simple, intermediate, or complex when describing procedures. **Simple** codes cover a single treatment area, one or two ports, and/or two or fewer simple blocks. **Intermediate** codes cover the treatment of two separate areas, three or more ports on a single treatment area, or three or more simple blocks. **Complex** codes cover three or more areas, custom blocking, tangential ports, wedge rotation beam, field-in-field, or other tissue compensation that does not meet IMRT guidelines.

Clinical Brachytherapy Procedures

Clinical brachytherapy is a form of radiation oncology that uses implanted radioelements, natural and artificial, to treat cancerous tissue. These implants are divided into two types: **sources,** which are permanently placed interstitially or inside a cavity; or **ribbons**, which are temporary implants. Like other radiation oncology procedures, brachytherapy uses a category system of simple, intermediate, and complex when describing procedures. **Simple** refers to the placement of 1–4 sources/ribbons, **intermediate** refers to the placement of 5–10 sources/ribbons, and **complex** applications are when more than 10 sources/ribbons are placed within the body. When coding these procedures, always note the **dose rate** and any **channels** that are mentioned in the procedure description.

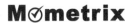

Nuclear Medicine Procedures

Nuclear medicine procedures are radiological services that involve the introduction of radioactive tracer substances into the body—inhaled, injected into the bloodstream, or ingested—to locate and diagnose diseases in various bodily systems. These types of procedures can be performed separately or in tandem with other procedures. These procedures do not include the actual **radiopharmaceuticals** (the radioactive substances used for the procedure) and drugs used in the procedure: When coding these procedures, include the supply code for the substances used. In addition, confirm the areas and types of imaging performed in the procedure's description.

Cardiovascular System

Typical nuclear medicine procedures performed on the cardiovascular system include **myocardial perfusion**, in which radioactive tracer substances flow through the blood that supplies the cardiac muscle; and **cardiac blood pool imaging**, which tracks how blood flows through the heart to the rest of the body. Several factors may impact the coding of these procedures. First, check the **type of procedure** performed, as usual. Next, check the **type of technique or scan** (such as a single-photon emission computerized tomography test or a first-pass technique) that is performed. In addition, note the **number of studies** performed during the procedure, because multiple studies can be performed during a single procedure.

Chapter Quiz

Ready to see how well you retained what you just read? Scan the QR code to go directly to the chapter quiz interface for this study guide. If you're using a computer, simply visit the bonus page at **mometrix.com/bonus948/cpc** and click the Chapter Quizzes link.

Laboratory and Pathology

Transform passive reading into active learning! After immersing yourself in this chapter, put your comprehension to the test by taking a quiz. The insights you gained will stay with you longer this way. Scan the QR code to go directly to the chapter quiz interface for this study guide. If you're using a computer, simply visit the bonus page at **mometrix.com/bonus948/cpc** and click the Chapter Quizzes link.

Laboratory and Pathology Procedures

Laboratory and pathology procedures cover various types of diagnostic lab work used in the diagnosis of diseases and conditions. Additionally, proprietary lab analyses (PLA) codes are provided to describe a single unique lab test commercially available in the United States for use on humans and made by a specific manufacturer or performed by a specific lab. These codes are covered in CPT code range **0001U** through **0363U**. Laboratory and pathology procedures are covered in CPT code range **80047** through **89398** and cover the following procedures:

- Organ- and disease-oriented panels
- Drug assays, both therapeutic and nontherapeutic
- Consultations on clinical pathology
- Urinalysis (testing urine)
- Molecular pathology (analysis of genetic material)
- Genomic sequencing
- Hematology and coagulation studies (testing blood)
- Immunology studies
- Transfusion medicine (tests used on donor blood)
- Microbiology studies (analysis of bacteria, viruses, and similar specimens)
- Anatomical and surgical pathology (inspecting cells and tissue taken from patients)
- Cytopathology and cytogenetic studies
- Reproductive medicine procedures

Organ and Disease Panels

Organ and disease panels are a type of procedure that analyzes and quantifies various chemicals and substances in a blood sample to provide information on metabolic functions and physical status. Each type of panel tests a number of different substances, such as albumin, glucose, potassium, sodium, urea nitrogen, and antibodies. When coding these procedures, it is important to select the code that contains as many substances listed in the procedure description as possible. If there's an overlap between two types of panels, choose the one that includes the largest number of listed substances and code the remainder as individual tests. In addition, pay attention to the specific substances listed in each panel because they may differ between similar panels. For instance, calcium is included in two types of basic metabolic panels, but one uses ionized calcium whereas the other uses total calcium.

Drug Testing

Types of Drug Testing Procedures

Drug assays are procedures used to detect the presence of drugs in the patient or subject's body, typically through blood, urine, or other bodily fluids or tissues. Drug assays are divided into two different types: **presumptive** and **definitive**. A presumptive drug procedure is used to identify the possible presence of a drug or a general class of drug in the subject's body. Meanwhile, a definitive drug procedure is used to determine a qualitative and/or quantitative value of a drug in the patient's system. It should be noted that, although both tests are often performed in sequence, a definitive test does not by definition require a presumptive test. Also, if the same procedure is performed on multiple specimen types from a single patient, then modifier 59 should be appended on each additional reported code.

Presumptive Drug Class Screening

Presumptive drug class screening procedures are used to identify the possible presence of a drug or a general class of drug in the subject's body. There are a few factors that must be taken into account when coding these types of procedures. The primary factor that defines the code selected is the **method of analysis**, whether by direct observation, such as a card or dipstick, or by chemical analysis, such as chromatography or mass spectrometry. These codes are only reported once, regardless of how many classes of drugs are tested for. Always check the procedure notes to determine what types of processes are used.

Definitive Drug Testing

Definitive drug testing procedures are used to identify specific classes of drugs, both in type and number, in a given patient's system. This process typically covers in-depth analysis, such as chromatography with mass spectrometry. The primary factor that defines the code selected is the **class of drug**, such as alcohols or skeletal muscle relaxants. An additional factor for some codes is the **number of analytes**. For example, the code for three or more alcohol biomarkers is different from the code for just one. Although some codes are meant for specific drugs, such as cocaine, other codes cover a generic class. For example, the drugs Paxil, Prozac, and Doxepin would fall under code 80335 because they're all cyclic antidepressants.

Therapeutic Drug Assays

Therapeutic drug assays are a type of drug testing procedure used to measure the presence and quantity of a specific prescribed medicine in the patient's system. This is done to monitor the levels of medical substances in order to keep the amount of drug within therapeutic levels and to prevent overdose or otherwise toxic side effects. This is typically performed on blood, blood serum, blood plasma, or CSF. These procedures are coded based on the **specific drug**, similar to definitive drug testing. Unlike with definitive drug testing, the number of metabolites or other units is not required to be known for code selection purposes.

Evocative/Suppression Testing

Medical Purpose

Evocative/suppression testing is a form of laboratory procedure designed to measure the release of certain bodily substances, enzymes, and hormones, such as corticotropin-releasing hormone or insulin. During the test, a particular enzyme, hormone, or other bodily substance is given an initial measurement. Then, additional substances are administered in order to elicit a response to determine if the levels are either suppressed or stimulated, after which the measurements are repeated and quantified. These procedures are often repeated multiple times. Evocative/suppression testing is typically performed to test for disorders of the endocrine system, such as human growth hormone deficiency, renal problems, or thyroid issues.

Coding

Evocative/suppression testing covers the laboratory procedures involved in the testing of certain bodily substances, enzymes, and hormones. Similar to organ and disease panels, each code includes multiple types of substance that are tested, although evocative/suppression tests typically have multiple iterations of each test. For example, an aldosterone suppression panel has two instances of aldosterone and two renin analyses. However, the individual tests themselves are not coded, so an aldosterone suppression panel would only use the single code 80408 as opposed to the four individual codes for the tests used. When reviewing the procedure notes, make sure that all iterations of each substance are mentioned and accounted for. These codes are for the actual testing procedure; for the administration of the actual evocative or suppressive substances, see codes **96365** through **96368** and **96372** through **96376**, located in the "Medicine" section of the CPT handbook.

Consultations

A clinical pathology consult is when a physician or other qualified healthcare provider requests the services, including written reports or information of the movement of drugs within the body, of a clinical pathologist in relation to tests and professional judgment. These procedures are distinct from a standard E/M consult because they do not involve the pathologist evaluating the patient. This does not include simply reporting test results. When coding these procedures, confirm whether the consultation did or did not include a **review of the patient's history and records**, because that defines the complexity of the consult. If the consult includes evaluating or examining a patient, see the relevant codes in the "E/M" section of CPT.

Urinalysis

Urinalysis is a set of laboratory procedures that revolve around the testing of a patient's urine. Although urinalysis is used in other procedures such as drug tests, the codes in the "Urinalysis" section of CPT focus on separately identifiable procedures, typically testing for substances in the urine such as glucose, hemoglobin, and protein; screening and culture of bacteria; or pregnancy tests that use urine. When coding these procedures, check the procedure notes for the specific **purpose** of the test. In addition, if the test is performed to check for substances, check the level of **automation** and the use of **microscopy**. If a specific analysis is being performed, refer to the appropriate subsection of the "Pathology and Laboratory" section.

Molecular Pathology

Procedures and Codes

Molecular pathology covers a number of laboratory procedures involving the analysis of deoxyribonucleic acid (DNA) and ribonucleic acid in order to detect various genetic disorders and related issues. This is done by analyzing a patient's genetic code for **germline** or **somatic** variations to see if the patient's genes do not match the normal sequence. Germline variations are inherited genetics, whereas somatic variations are singular mutations that aren't passed down. This section also includes tests for **human leukocyte antigens**, which are the protein markers that help regulate the immune system. Codes in this section include all of the analytic services involved in performing the tests, and they are divided into tiers based on how commonly the procedure is performed.

Tier 1 Molecular Pathology Procedures

Tier 1 molecular pathology procedures are a set of molecular pathology procedures from **81170** through **81383** that are commonly performed. These codes represent gene-specific procedures that cover a wide variety of common genetic disorders, such as fragile X syndrome, cystic fibrosis, sickle cell anemia, hereditary nonpolyposis colorectal cancer, and other issues. Procedure codes are defined by the specific sequence, or **analyte**, that they cover, and they include a list of **associated disorders** or conditions that are being tested for. Several codes will focus on a **specific type of analysis**. For example, 81223 is a full gene sequence analysis cystic fibrosis transmembrane conductance regulator. When reviewing the procedure notes for these codes, check for any other details of the analysis that may be mentioned.

Tier 2 Molecular Pathology Procedures

Tier 2 molecular pathology procedures include a variety of molecular pathology procedures that are uncommon or rare compared to the procedures listed in Tier 1. Although medically necessary, the procedures used are performed at lower rates due to a relative scarcity of the disease being tested for. Unlike Tier 1 procedures, Tier 2 procedures are grouped by the **level** of analysis required, like a Level 7 procedure that covers an 11 to 25 exon DNA sequence analysis, as well as the specific sequence being analyzed. Each code covers a wide variety of analysis procedures, listed alphabetically by analyte, so procedure notes should always be checked for the specific procedure. If the specific analyte is not covered by either Tier 1 or Tier 2, then code **81479** (for unlisted molecular pathology procedure) should be used instead.

Genomic Sequencing Procedures (GSPs)

Genomic sequencing procedures (GSPs) are a type of molecular pathology procedure in which multiple genes or genetic regions are tested and analyzed for medically significant issues. Unlike standard molecular pathology procedures, GSPs are used to cover a large number of related genes and sequences that may contribute to a condition. They can be applied to both germline and **neoplastic** (abnormal or cancerous) samples, and they are reapplied when new information is obtained. This section also includes related molecular techniques, such as the polymerase chain reaction, which are used for analysis. These procedures cover a wide variety of genetic disorders, such as those related to Ashkenazi Jew-associated disorders or hereditary cardiomyopathy.

Coding

Genomic sequencing and related procedure codes are listed by the class of issues that are covered by the procedure, such as fetal chromosomal aneuploidy or hearing loss. Each procedure covers several gene sequences that must be included in the assay. For example, code 81437 must include MAX, SDHB, SDHC, SDHD, TMEM127, and VHL in the procedure description. If an assay uses genes that are covered by multiple procedure codes, pick the most specific for the disorder being reported. Also, if only some of the gene groups are tested, but not all required gene sequences are included, report the individual codes from Tier 1 or Tier 2, or use code 81479 if the test is unlisted.

Multianalyte Assays with Algorithmic Analysis (MAAA) Procedures

Multianalyte assays with algorithmic analysis (MAAA) procedures are specific types of laboratory and pathology procedures that combine multiple molecular and biochemical assays, patient demographics, and other clinical information into an algorithm to predict the likelihood of or risk for a disease or condition occurring in a patient. The inclusion of additional data, such as medical records and other laboratory tests, differentiates these tests from GSPs and similar multianalyte assays. MAAA procedures include the disease type, the materials analyzed and markers used, the methodology, the specimen, the algorithm result, and the type of report. These codes include all of the analytic services necessary to perform the procedure, in addition to the algorithmic analysis.

Coding

MAAA procedures are listed initially by the **type of condition** that's being tested for, such as coronary artery disease or fetal congenital abnormalities. If there's a general type of condition being examined, like cancer, always confirm the specific type of condition, such as "cancer (ovarian)." If there is no additional type listed, check the **analytes being analyzed** to clarify the procedure.

Not all MAAA procedures are in the "Pathology and Laboratory" section. If a procedure is not listed in that section, check **Appendix O** of the CPT book for additional codes. If the procedure is in neither location, report it using procedure code **81599.**

Chemistry

Chemistry procedures in CPT cover the chemical analysis of body tissue or fluid specimens derived from a patient. These codes are used for the detection of specific substances that may be difficult to locate via visual inspection, such as occult blood in the feces or cholesterol in the blood. Chemistry codes are organized by the **specific analyte** being tested, such as ammonia, blood gases, or glucose, and they may be subdivided in certain cases by their **method of analysis** (such as qualitative or quantitative) or **subtype** (such as fetal chemical hemoglobin). Review the procedure notes to determine the most specific test code to report. These procedures are considered separate from a panel of tests, such as an organ- or disease-oriented panel.

Hematology and Coagulation

Hematology and coagulation procedures cover laboratory and pathological examinations of a patient's blood, such as bleeding time, clotting factor tests, coagulation time, and viscosity. Codes in this section are divided by the **specific procedure** being performed, although some procedures are broken down into subtypes based on the **category of the procedure**, such as clotting tests for factor II or factor VIII. These procedures may be included in certain panels or MAAA procedures. These codes only cover blood testing procedures; for procedures such as blood banking procedures or tests for agglutinins, refer to the respective sections in CPT.

Immunology

Immunology procedures are laboratory and pathology procedures that involve the human immune system and its various chemical and cellular components, such as antibody identification or counting the various types of white blood cells. Codes in this section are divided by the **specific procedure**, but they may be subdivided depending on the **analyte being analyzed**. For example, a total count of T cells has a different code from when a T cell count with absolute CD4 and CD8 count with ratio is performed. These procedures do not cover the analysis of specific antibodies, and they are meant to cover a comparatively general testing methodology.

Qualitative Immunoassay

A qualitative immunoassay is a subset of immunology procedures involving the type and relative number of antibodies related to specific infectious diseases in the patient's blood. This also includes tests for human immunodeficiency virus (HIV). Codes in this section are divided by the **specific disease** antibodies that are being tested for, such as *Giardia lamblia* or influenza. When coding these procedures, code as specifically as possible according to the procedural notes. If multiple assays are performed for different classes of immunoglobulin, then each assay must be coded separately, despite testing for the same disease. These codes are for lengthy, multiple-step methods of antibody detection; use code 86318 for single-step and related methods.

Tissue Typing

Tissue typing is a form of immunological procedure that focuses on the compatibility of tissues and organs from differing sources. These procedures are typically performed prior to organ and tissue transplants in order to determine compatibility and hopefully avoid tissue rejection and similar issues. Typically, a specific tissue typing procedure is only done once, and it is recorded for all instances of transplantation involving the patient. These codes are divided by the **specific procedure**, although some have subtypes based on the specific methodology (e.g., multiple antigens vs. a single antigen). The recipient of the transplant and the original donor or donors should be coded for the procedures performed.

Transfusions

Transfusion medicine is a category of laboratory and pathology procedures that covers the transfusion of blood and blood components, such as plasma or leukocytes, between individual sources. This section covers a variety of procedures, including antibody tests, blood typing (including paternity tests), screening for antigens, and storing of frozen blood. These codes are divided by the **specific procedure**, although some (such as blood typing) have related codes based on methodology or additional processes. These codes are for diagnostic and storage procedures; procedures such as apheresis and therapeutic phlebotomy are found elsewhere in CPT and should be coded appropriately.

Microbiology

Microbiology procedures in CPT involve the analysis, identification, and culturing of microorganisms for the purposes of diagnosing disorders or diseases. These procedures cover a number of specialties, including **bacteriology** (the study of bacteria), **mycology** (the study of fungi), **parasitology** (the study of parasites), and **virology** (the study of viruses). Codes in this section are initially categorized by the **specific procedure**, although many codes have subcategories determined by the **methodology**, such as different analysis techniques; or the **sample source** used in the analysis or culture. These codes are meant for presumptive identification; more definitive tests require additional tests and should be coded separately. If multiple specimens are used for a test, append modifier 59 to the code. If the same test is performed multiple times on the same sample on the same day, append modifier 91 to the code.

Primary Source Microbiology

Primary source microbiology procedures involve the analysis, detection, and culturing of specific infectious agents. These codes are used when the type of virus, bacteria, or other pathogen is known, either categorically (such as an adenovirus) or specifically (such as herpes simplex virus type 1). These codes are organized initially by **method of detection** and then by **general classification** of the particular pathogen. The general codes also have several subcategories based on the **specific type** of pathogen. If the specific type of infectious agent is not known, report the general methodology code as the most specific code selectable (e.g., "Not otherwise specified, each organism").

Anatomical Pathology

Anatomical pathology procedures in CPT are primarily **autopsy** procedures, also known as **necropsy** procedures, which involve the examination of a dead body by a trained physician. These codes are organized by type and level of detail: **gross**, **gross and microscopic**, **regional**, and **forensic examination**. Gross examination involves physical and visual examination of the deceased. Microscopic examination involves taking tissue samples for additional analysis. Regional autopsies cover a single bodily system or organ. Forensic autopsies are performed in the event of a criminal investigation, and they may or may not include a coroner's call of whether the death was natural, accidental, or deliberate. All codes are assumed to be performed by the physician on site; if an outside lab performs the service, use modifier 90 in conjunction with the appropriate code.

Cytopathology

Cytopathology procedures are pathology procedures that involve the study, analysis, and diagnosis of diseases at a cellular level, typically through the microscopic study of fragmented bodily tissue and free cells from the patient's body. Such samples can be acquired either through manual removal (such as with a wash or a needle) or through spontaneous exfoliation of cells. This also includes forensic cytopathology and DNA analysis procedures. This typically involves the removal of cells through various means for study and analysis. Cytopathology procedure codes are categorized primarily by the **technique** used to analyze the samples provided, such as in situ hybridization. Gynecological cytopathology procedures are coded separately from more generalized cytopathology procedures.

Gynecological

This section of cytopathology procedures focuses primarily on **gynecological** procedures, or procedures involving the female reproductive system. Typically, these codes will involve acquiring samples from the cervix or vagina for study and screening. These procedures are organized primarily by the **method of screening**, such as manual screening or automated thin layer preparation, although several procedures will have related codes that cover rescreening by the physician. In addition, check the procedural notes to see if the **Bethesda system**, a system for reporting pap smear results, is used during the procedure, because that will alter the code selection per the notes in CPT.

Cytogenetic Studies

Cytogenetic studies are a form of molecular pathology procedures that study the relationship between **chromosomes**, the DNA molecules that contain genetic material, and diseases or conditions. These procedures involve analysis of chromosomes via visual or molecular means, as well as procedures for storing and preserving cells for later examination. Codes in this section are organized by the **specific procedure** (for storage) or **method of analysis.** Several codes use the **number of cells counted** in order to narrow down the code selection. These codes should not be used to report procedures used as part of an MAAA procedure or as part of a molecular pathology procedure; only use these codes if the cytogenetic study is being performed on its own.

Surgical Pathology

Gross and Microscopic Examination Procedures

Gross and microscopic examination procedures are surgical pathology procedures that involve the analysis of tissue specimens taken from a patient for the purposes of examination and diagnosis. Examination codes are divided into **gross only** and **gross and microscopic** examinations. Gross exams include a visual inspection of the specimen, whereas gross and microscopic exams include a detailed look at the specimen under a microscope. Procedure codes related to examination are separated into levels in CPT, with Level I representing gross examination of any tissue specimen and all of the other levels representing gross and microscopic examination of various categories of tissues. If multiple specimens of the same type are taken from a single patient, then each specimen is coded as an individual, not as a group.

Procedures and Coding

Surgical pathology covers not just gross and microscopic examination of tissue samples taken from patients; additional procedure codes are given for specialized and non-microscopic analysis and examination, such as histochemical stains, morphometric analysis, and macroscopic examination and dissection. It also covers additional related procedures, such as consultations and reports on prepared tissues. Codes in this portion of the "Surgical Pathology" section are ordered by the **specific procedure**, and they often include add-on codes for procedures that may require **multiple specimens or procedures.** Always check for parentheticals underneath each procedure description because several codes may not be reported in conjunction with others located elsewhere in CPT.

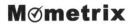

In Vivo Procedures

In vivo and miscellaneous laboratory procedures are procedures, typically noninvasive, that involve the analysis of bodily fluids or substances such as bilirubin, hemoglobin, urine, feces, sputum, and sweat to assess, quantify, or detect certain values or substances. These procedures are sufficiently different from other laboratory procedures that they are placed in a separate category to differentiate them. In vivo procedures are organized based on the **specific fluid or substance** (such as bilirubin or hemoglobin) that is being analyzed, whereas miscellaneous procedures are organized based on the **procedure** and the **substance being tested for** (such as leukocytes or fat).

Reproductive Medicine Procedures

Reproductive medicine procedures are laboratory procedures that revolve around reproductive cells and tissues, particularly oocytes, nonimplanted embryos, and sperm. These procedures cover the analysis and identification of various reproductive cells, as well as artificial insemination and short- or long-term cryopreservation of embryos, oocytes, sperm, and reproductive tissue for later use or analysis. Procedures in this category are organized by **specific procedure** (such as cryopreservation), with additional codes related to **quantity** (in the case of fertilization or biopsy), the **specific analysis type**, or the **type of tissue being preserved** (in the case of cryopreservation). Cryopreservation and storage codes, unless otherwise specified, cover all units from a specific patient being preserved or stored.

Proprietary Laboratory Analysis

Proprietary laboratory analysis procedures are special procedures that either can only be performed by a single laboratory, or are owned by a specific brand or organization and licensed to multiple providing laboratories. These procedures cover a wide variety of analysis procedures, such as MAAA and GSP, but they do not technically fall into those categories due to their proprietary nature. These codes are easily identified by a "U" in the procedure code's fifth character space; there is a list of proprietary names located in **Appendix O** of the CPT handbook. Codes in this section are only reported if the type of analysis performed matches the code descriptor and falls under the proprietary name listed in **Appendix O**.

Chapter Quiz

Ready to see how well you retained what you just read? Scan the QR code to go directly to the chapter quiz interface for this study guide. If you're using a computer, simply visit the bonus page at mometrix.com/bonus948/cpc and click the Chapter Quizzes link.

Medicine

Transform passive reading into active learning! After immersing yourself in this chapter, put your comprehension to the test by taking a quiz. The insights you gained will stay with you longer this way. Scan the QR code to go directly to the chapter quiz interface for this study guide. If you're using a computer, simply visit the bonus page at **mometrix.com/bonus948/cpc** and click the Chapter Quizzes link.

Immunizations

Immune Globulins, Serum, and Recombinant Products

The immune globulins, serum, and recombinant products subcategory contains a list of codes used for substances derived from blood created for the purposes of immunization. These include **immune globulins** and **serum**, which are typically derived from human blood, and **recombinant products**, which are produced via a mix of genetically altered human- and animal-sourced blood products and proteins. Codes for these products are organized by the **specific substance or disease** that the globulin, serum, or recombinant is designed to protect against, and they are meant to be used in conjunction with the appropriate administration procedure codes. For administration procedures, see codes **90460** through **0173A**, located later in the "Medicine" section of CPT.

Administration Procedures

Immunization administration procedures are used when a specific vaccine or toxoid is administered to a patient to generate an immune response. These codes cover the actual procedure of administering a vaccine and may be used in conjunction with vaccine and toxoid product codes if the office, facility, or hospital doing the administration also supplied the vaccine or toxoid. The codes are divided into three categories: administration with counseling (**90460**), administration via injection (**90471**), and administration via intranasal or oral route (**90473**), each with add-on codes for extra vaccines. Other codes are listed in this section identifying the age of the patient or disease being prevented. Each additional vaccine administered is reported separately. These codes are reported separately from E/M codes if performed in conjunction with those services.

Vaccine and Toxoid Products

Vaccine and toxoid product codes are used to code the actual vaccines or toxoids that are administered during immunization procedures. Because these codes do not describe actual procedures, they should not be reported without the appropriate immunization procedure code, nor should they be reported with modifier 51 if multiple instances of a vaccine are used. These codes are organized by the **type of disease or toxoid** that the vaccine is meant to immunize the patient from. If a patient is given a combination vaccine for multiple pathogens, then the appropriate combination vaccine code should be reported instead of the individual separate vaccine codes; for example, do not report the hepatitis A and B vaccines separately if a combination hepatitis A and B immunization is given.

Psychiatry

Interactive Complexity

Psychiatric procedures may be complicated by the patient's condition, characteristics, or situational factors that disrupt or interfere with communication between the provider and the subject. In CPT, this is termed "interactive complexity." Typically, these factors may occur if a patient has a third party (such as a guardian, parole officer, child welfare agent, or an accompanying family member or interpreter) with them during the service. According to CPT, interactive complexity is reported as an add-on code to a diagnostic psychiatric evaluation, psychotherapy, and group psychotherapy when one or more of the following is demonstrated:

- Management of maladaptive communication
- Emotions or behaviors that interfere with a caregiver's understanding or ability to assist
- Evidence, disclosure, or discussion of an event that requires a mandated report
- Use of tools, interpreters, or translators to communicate with a patient who has difficulty speaking or understanding

Psychotherapy Procedures

Psychotherapy procedures are medical procedures meant to treat a patient's mental illness or behavioral issues. These typically include things like communication, helping to alleviate emotional disturbance, altering destructive or otherwise maladaptive behaviors, and encouraging positive mental development. Psychotherapy procedures are organized by the **time spent** with the patient. In addition, this section includes add-on codes used in conjunction with E/M procedures performed as part of the psychotherapy procedure. If this is done, the E/M services and psychotherapy services should be separately identifiable and distinct. These codes are meant for single patients, not for family procedures.

Psychotherapy for Crisis

Psychotherapy for crisis is a psychiatric procedure meant for patients that are in a state of acute mental and psychological distress, such as a mental breakdown, severe anxiety attack, display of suicidal intent, or other extreme moments of crisis. This includes urgent assessment, treatment, and the mobilization of any resources needed to safely defuse the crisis and minimize emotional or psychological trauma. These codes are used to report the first 30 to 74 minutes of intervention involving the patient and any family members present, with an add-on code for each 30-minute block afterward. If fewer than 30 minutes are spent during the psychotherapy for crisis, CPT states that codes **90832** or **90833** (if E/M are performed) should be reported instead.

Dialysis

Hemodialysis

Hemodialysis is a type of medical procedure that uses a machine to artificially filter waste and excess water from the patient's blood in the place of their kidneys, typically as part of a treatment for renal disease or damage. These procedures include E/M procedures related to the disease on the day of dialysis. The procedures are separated based on whether a physician or other qualified professional performs a single evaluation, repeated evaluation, or an access flow study during the dialysis process. CPT reveals that these codes are used for inpatient procedures and outpatient, non-ESRD (end-stage renal disease) services.

End-Stage Renal Disease (ESRD) Services

End-stage renal disease (ESRD) services are dialysis procedures performed in an outpatient setting for an individual in the terminal stages of renal disease, when the kidneys are essentially nonfunctional. These age-specific procedures include the establishment of a dialysis schedule, outpatient E/M services, and patient management, and they are reported once a month. Codes in this section are organized primarily by the **age of the patient** and then by the **number of face-to-face visits** performed by a healthcare professional per month. Alternatively, if ESRD services are provided for less than a full month, use codes **90967** through **90970** with a number of units equal to the number of days.

Ophthalmology

General Ophthalmology Services

General ophthalmology services are procedures in which an ophthalmologist provides general vision care services for a patient, which typically involve nonspecialized treatment, examinations, and other general diagnostic procedures. General services are organized primarily by whether a patient is **new** or **established**, based on E/M guidelines. After that, procedures are based on whether the services are **intermediate** or **comprehensive**. Intermediate services, as defined by CPT, are the evaluation of a new or existing condition that's been complicated by a new condition or problem. Comprehensive services, by contrast, are defined by CPT as a general examination and evaluation of the entire visual system.

Special Ophthalmology Services

Special ophthalmology services cover ophthalmology procedures that go beyond the requirements of general services or involve a special treatment or evaluation of the visual system. These services may be reported either in addition to general ophthalmology procedures or as part of a patient's E/M services. These codes include the interpretation and reporting of the results, and they may or may not include the technical component of the procedure. Procedures under this category are organized by the **specific procedure** that is being performed, such as computerized corneal topography or a visual field examination. Note any parentheticals under the procedure descriptions for alternative codes or codes that may not be used in conjunction with the selected procedure code.

Otorhinolaryngological Services

Special otorhinolaryngological services are diagnostic and treatment procedures involving the ear, nose, and throat that exceed the scope of standard E/M services or outpatient consultation. These can include speech tests, vestibular function tests, evaluations of cochlear implants, and other related procedures. Codes in this section are organized by the **specific category of procedure**, such as vestibular function tests or evaluative and therapeutic services, and they are then organized by the **specific procedure type**. When coding these procedures, always check any parentheticals underneath the procedure's description for alternative codes or codes that should not be reported in conjunction with that procedure.

Cardiovascular

Coronary Therapeutic Services

Coronary therapeutic service codes cover procedures meant to repair or relieve either temporary or chronic occlusion of a blood vessel. CPT describes these procedures as **percutaneous coronary intervention** procedures. These procedures include, in order of difficulty, coronary stents, percutaneous transluminal coronary angioplasties, and atherectomies, and they are performed on major coronary arteries, coronary artery branches, and coronary artery bypasses. Procedures in this section are organized by the **type of procedure** being performed, and they are accompanied by add-on codes indicating additional coronary branches or arteries that the procedures are performed on.

Echocardiography

Echocardiography is a procedure in which images of the heart or great vessels are obtained via ultrasound scanning equipment, typically with real-time imaging, documentation of Doppler signals, or both. These procedures may be performed at rest, as part of a cardiovascular stress test, or both. These codes are organized by the chosen **method of approach** (either transthoracic or transesophageal), then by the **types of imaging** that are used during the scan (such as a spectral

Doppler echocardiography), and finally by whether the procedure is part of a **stress test**. Procedures in this section include the interpretation and documentation of the scan's results.

Cardiac Catheterization

Cardiac catheterization procedures are a type of diagnostic procedure involving the insertion and positioning of a **catheter** (a long, thin tube) for the purposes of analyzing blood flow, intracardiac and intravascular pressure, blood oxygen saturation, and other information. These procedures can be performed on both sides or on either side of the heart (left or right), and they are typically performed on patients with congenital heart disease or other heart-related issues. These procedures are organized based on the **procedure** being performed (left, right, or combined left and right heart catheterization or angiography), although many codes (**93455** through **93461**) are additional codes for coronary angiography (code **93454**).

Pulmonary and Allergy

Pulmonary Diagnostic Testing and Therapy

Pulmonary diagnostic testing and therapy covers procedures that involve diagnostic analysis and treatment of the lungs and pulmonary system, including analysis of air flow, lung volume, pulmonary function, and other data, as well as inhalation treatments with aerosolized medication. These procedures are organized by the **specific procedure**, and they include all of the necessary laboratory procedures and interpretation of results by a physician. Always check the parentheticals under each procedure description for alternative codes and for codes that may not be reported in conjunction with the specific procedure. These procedures may be performed in conjunction with E/M procedures; if so, then report the appropriate code in conjunction with the codes in this section.

Allergen Immunotherapy Procedures

Allergen immunotherapy is a type of medical procedure in which a patient is slowly desensitized to environmental allergens to strengthen the patient's immune system and reduce harmful responses by means of an injection of allergenic extracts as antigens. For these procedures, the proper code can be determined if the procedure notes discuss whether the immunotherapy is only administered (in the case of codes **95115** and **95117**), if professional services for allergen immunotherapy are rendered in conjunction with an administration (in the case of codes **95120** through **95134**), or if the immunotherapy is only prepared and not administered to the patient (in the case of codes **95144** through **95170**). In addition, specific types of immunotherapies, such as insect venom, should be considered. In all cases, care should be taken to review the procedural notes provided.

Neurology and Central Nervous System

Sleep Medicine Testing

Sleep medicine covers procedures used to evaluate pediatric and adult patients for issues involving or occurring during the sleep cycle, such as sleep apnea or insomnia. These services are primarily diagnostic, and they include recording, interpreting, and reporting data as part of the procedure. Codes in this section are organized primarily by the **procedure performed**, and they are further subdivided by **any additional analysis performed** as a part of the study (e.g., respiratory analysis during a sleep study) or by the **age of the participant** in certain cases. If a study has fewer than 6 hours recorded during the procedure, append modifier 52 to the appropriate code.

Central Nervous System Assessments

Central nervous system assessments are medical tests meant to examine a patient's sensory neurons and cognitive functions to see if the nervous system is somehow impaired or underdeveloped. These assessments include memory and language, visual and auditory, and abstract reasoning skills testing. Procedures in this section are divided by the **specific type of assessment**, such as aphasia or neurobehavioral status examination, and they are further subdivided by the **time taken** during the procedure. For these codes, each given block of time (such as 1 hour or 30 minutes) counts as a single unit for the purposes of coding. For example, if an aphasia assessment takes 2 hours, the proper code to report would be 96105 × 2.

Hydration Procedures

Hydration procedures involve the intravenous injection of fluids, typically a mix of saline, dextrose, electrolytes, and other fluids. This can be performed to help a patient suffering from dehydration or nutrient deficiency recover quickly, or it can be performed with an included mixture of therapeutic or diagnostic medicine as part of a treatment program. These procedures are organized by the **time spent** during the procedure, typically in 1-hour blocks after the initial introduction. It should be noted that, in the case of hydration without drug infusion, the minimum time for infusion is 30 minutes. Infusions shorter than this should not be reported. For shorter times involving the introduction of drugs or other therapeutic substances, see code **96372** for injections.

Chemotherapy Procedures

Chemotherapy is a procedure in which highly complex **antineoplastic** (anticancer) drugs or other biological agents are administered to a patient for the purposes of treatment, typically for the purposes of destroying malignant lesions or tumors. Chemotherapy can be introduced by several methods: intravenously; via intramuscular injection directly into the lesion or lesions; or via various intra-arterial means. These procedures are organized by the **method of introduction** (intravenous or intra-arterial), and then either by the **number of lesions** (for intralesional) or the **length of infusion**, with add-on codes for time intervals greater than 30 minutes. The codes for the specific drugs should be coded separately because these codes only cover the actual administration of the treatment.

Photodynamic Therapy

Photodynamic therapy is a type of dermatological procedure used to treat cancerous and noncancerous lesions of the skin and related tissue via photosensitive drugs. After the drugs are applied, high-intensity light is used to activate the drugs, which then destroy the cells of any tissue that the drugs are applied to. The main procedures are organized by whether the treatment is **performed by a physician** or not. In addition, the section includes add-on codes for photodynamic therapy used for treating internal lesions, such as in the lungs or gastrointestinal system. These add-on codes are differentiated by the **duration of treatment**, and they should be reported in addition to the appropriate bronchoscopy or endoscopy codes.

Special Dermatological Procedures

Special dermatological procedures are miscellaneous procedures involving diagnostic analysis and treatment of skin issues. These include procedures such as ultraviolet light therapy, laser treatment of psoriasis, and reflectance confocal microscopy, as well as otherwise unlisted dermatological procedures. Because these procedures do not fit in with other procedural categories, they are filed under this category. Codes in this category are organized by **type of procedure**. Codes for reflectance confocal microscopy have several additional codes that are used to better report this procedure, in addition to add-on codes for each additional lesion that the procedure is performed on.

Physical Medicine and Rehabilitation

Physical medicine and rehabilitation procedures cover a specific type of medical evaluation used for physical therapy, occupational therapy, and athletic training evaluations. Similar to standard E/M procedures, physical medicine and rehabilitation codes typically include an assessment that contains medical history, an examination of systems, and clinical decision-making, and they list a typical amount of time spent on face-to-face contact with the providing physician. However, there are differences: Physical therapy requires a clinical presentation of changing characteristics, while occupational therapy assesses issues that may impede work. Codes in this section are first separated into the **type of evaluation** and then by the **level of complexity** (e.g., low, medium, or high). Each procedure requires that all components must be included to be accurately coded, regardless of patient status.

Modalities

Modalities, as referred to in this section of CPT, refer to a variety of therapeutic methods that attempt to produce positive changes in a patient's condition. These procedures are typically noninvasive, and they cover things such as heat and cold packs, electrostimulation, or exposure to infrared or ultraviolet light. Modalities are divided into **supervised** procedures, which do not require direct contact with the patient, and **constant attendance**, which does require direct contact with the patient. These procedures are listed by the **specific method** used. In the case of modalities requiring constant attendance, codes are listed in units of 15 minutes. For example, a 30-minute contrast bath would be coded as 97034 twice.

Therapeutic Procedures

Therapeutic procedures cover a wide variety of physical, social, and psychological services aimed at improving a patient's physical, cognitive, or social functionality. In addition to physical exercises and manipulation, therapeutic procedures also include forms of training, such as wheelchair use and community integration training, that allow the patient to work or interact with others. These procedures require direct contact between the patient and the provider. Procedures in this category are grouped by the **specific procedure**, and they are often listed in units of time (typically in blocks of 15 minutes). For example, 1 hour of gait training would be coded as four instances of code 97116.

Acupuncture

Acupuncture procedures are a form of alternative medicine that involves the insertion of needles into key positions on the body for relief of certain symptoms. The insertion of the needles may also be accompanied by a mild electrical stimulation via a current run through the needles. Acupuncture services are reported in units of 15 minutes, and they are organized depending on whether the procedure does or does not use **electrical stimulation** through the needles. When reporting, the code for an initial procedure is only used once per day; multiple instances of treatment should be counted via add-on codes.

Osteopathic and Chiropractic Manipulation Procedures

Osteopathic and chiropractic procedures are a form of alternative medicine involving the manipulation of body parts for relief of pain, stiffness, and certain other symptoms. Osteopathic manipulation treatment involves the manipulation of muscles and bones, whereas chiropractic manipulation treatment involves the manipulation of the spinal column. These procedures are organized by the **number of bodily regions** that are manipulated by the provider, and they typically include a pre-manipulation assessment of the patient. A list of bodily regions used for osteopathic manipulation treatment and chiropractic manipulation treatment procedures is provided in the relevant sections. If the provider performs E/M services on the patient, code them separately from the actual osteopathic and chiropractic procedures.

Patient Education and Training

Education and training procedures cover educational and instruction services prescribed and provided by a qualified health professional to a nonqualified individual, such as the patient, patient's guardian, or caregiver, for the purpose of treating an established illness or minimizing or delaying further issues. These procedures are different from the counseling and education provided as part of an E/M service because they typically involve education beyond what such a service would entail. Procedures of this type are organized by the **number of individual patients or caregivers** that undergo education, and they are coded in blocks of 30 minutes. These services are meant for individuals; for group training, see code **99078.**

Non-Face-to-Face Services

Non-face-to-face services are a type of patient assessment, separate from E/M, that takes place over a long distance between a qualified healthcare professional and a patient or their guardian or caregiver. These types of services can be performed either over the telephone or via online communications, the latter of which must include recording and permanent storage of the encounter. Codes related to these procedures are organized by the **method of communication**, either telephone or online. Codes for telephone communications are determined by the total amount of time spent in medical discussion. The codes for telephone communication are not reported if the communication leads to a face-to-face encounter within 24 hours or the nearest available urgent appointment.

Moderate Sedation

Activities Involved in Moderate Sedation Services

Moderate sedation, also known as **conscious sedation**, is a form of anesthesia in which a patient remains conscious enough to respond to verbal or tactile commands, while able to breathe on their own without assistance. These sorts of procedures differ from MAC in that the physicians themselves perform the sedation instead of a separate anesthesiologist. Moderate sedation services include **preservice, intraservice**, and **postservice** work. Preservice includes assessment of the patient's history, allergies, and vital signs before sedation. Intraservice work begins with the actual administration of the sedation, and it is used to determine the proper CPT code to be used. Finally, postservice work includes postsedation assessments and readiness for discharge.

Procedures and Coding

Moderate sedation procedures are identified by the lack of an anesthesiologist or certified registered nurse anesthesiologist performing the actual procedure; instead, the physicians themselves provide the sedation service. These codes are primarily organized by whether an **independent trained observer** is present to assist in monitoring the patient's level of consciousness and physical status. Codes are further separated by the **age of the patient**, with 5 years old being the dividing line. Codes indicate the amount of intraservice time in blocks of 15 minutes. For example, if a 6-year-old patient undergoes moderate sedation with observation for 45 minutes, then the proper codes to report would be 99152 once and 99153 twice.

Chapter Quiz

Ready to see how well you retained what you just read? Scan the QR code to go directly to the chapter quiz interface for this study guide. If you're using a computer, simply visit the bonus page at **mometrix.com/bonus948/cpc** and click the Chapter Quizzes link.

International Classification of Diseases, 10th Revision, Clinical Modification (ICD-10-CM)

Transform passive reading into active learning! After immersing yourself in this chapter, put your comprehension to the test by taking a quiz. The insights you gained will stay with you longer this way. Scan the QR code to go directly to the chapter quiz interface for this study guide. If you're using a computer, simply visit the bonus page at **mometrix.com/bonus948/cpc** and click the Chapter Quizzes link.

Structure of ICD-10-CM Codes

Unlike CPT, ICD-10-CM codes consist of a set of up to seven characters and a decimal point that indicate the position of the diagnosis in ICD-10-CM. Generally speaking, ICD-10-CM codes are structured as follows:

- Each code begins with a **letter**, indicating the general category of the code in the tabular list. For example, L is for a skin condition.
- After the letter are **two numbers**, which further narrow the code's position in the listing and general type of condition. For example, L02 is for a cutaneous abscess.
- The first three characters are followed by a **decimal point** to separate the general category from the specifics.
- The **fourth character** is used to narrow the diagnosis further. For example, L02.2 is for a cutaneous abscess of the trunk.
- The **fifth and sixth characters** provide the most specific diagnosis. For example, L02.211 is for a cutaneous abscess of the abdominal wall.
- A **seventh character** is typically used for additional information, such as the time of the encounter.
- If there are missing characters between the rest of the code and the seventh character, a **placeholder "X"** is used in place of the missing characters (e.g., M48.40**X**A).

ICD-10-CM Tabular List

The color-coded tabular list makes up the bulk of the ICD-10-CM coding book. The tabular list contains all of the diagnosis codes that have been officially added to ICD-10-CM, and it is arranged into sections based on general anatomical category or similar commonalities. The tabular list contains the following sections:

- **A through B**: Infectious and parasitic diseases
- **C through D49**: Neoplasms (e.g., cancer)
- **D50 through D89**: Blood, blood-forming organs, and certain immune disorders
- **E**: Endocrine, nutritional, and metabolic diseases
- **F**: Mental, behavioral, and neurodevelopmental disorders
- **G**: Nervous system
- **H (H00 through H59)**: Eye and adnexa
- **H (H60 through H95)**: Ear and mastoid process

- **I:** Circulatory system
- **J**: Respiratory system
- **K:** Digestive system
- **L:** Skin and subcutaneous tissue
- **M:** Musculoskeletal system and connective tissue
- **N:** Genitourinary system (male and female)
- **O:** Pregnancy, childbirth, and the **puerperium** (six weeks post childbirth)
- **P:** Conditions originating in the **perinatal** (immediately before and after birth) period
- **Q**: Congenital malformations, deformations, and chromosomal abnormalities
- **R:** Symptoms, signs, and abnormal findings
- **S through T:** Injury and poisoning
- **V through Y:** Factors influencing health status and contact with health services

Selecting the Correct ICD-10-CM Diagnosis Code

The ICD-10-CM coding book is used to code the condition that the patient is diagnosed with, based on the procedural notes provided. Although some diagnoses, such as cancer, injury, or poison, require additional or alternative steps, the vast majority of diagnosis code selection involves the following steps:

1. **Look up the diagnosis in the index.** The index lists all the diagnoses provided in ICD-10-CM in alphabetical order by the name of the condition, with indented subcategories listed underneath for more specific diagnoses. For example, a diagnosis of type 2 diabetes with polyneuropathy would be listed under **"Diabetes,"** followed by **"type 2, with,"** and then **"polyneuropathy."**
2. **Follow the code listed in the index to the proper code in the tabular list.** Once the condition is found in the index, follow the given code to the location in the tabular list. **Do not just use the code given in the index**; some codes are incomplete or may require additional characters.
3. **Report the codes in the proper sequence.** When coding diagnoses, the proper sequence is the order in which the conditions are mentioned in the procedural notes unless stated otherwise in ICD-10-CM.

Coding Neoplasm Diagnoses Using ICD-10-CM

Unlike other conditions, neoplasms (abnormal cell growth, such as a tumor) have a separate section within the ICD-10-CM book. Neoplasms are listed in a special table based on their anatomical location, with subcategories for more precise locations. For example, a neoplasm in the transverse colon would be found under **"intestine,"** then **"large, colon,"** and **"transverse."** ICD-10-CM also divides neoplasm codes by their behavior, which falls into six categories:

1. **Malignant primary**, where a cancer has spread from
2. **Malignant secondary**, where a cancer has spread to
3. **Carcinoma in situ**, for a malignant mass isolated to a single place
4. **Benign**, for noncancerous neoplasms
5. **Uncertain behavior**, for neoplasms whose behavior has not yet been identified
6. **Unspecified behavior**, for neoplasms whose behavior is not outlined in the procedural notes

Many neoplasm codes will be found in sections C and D of the tabular list. Always check the code in the tabular list after locating it in the index.

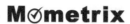

Coding Injury Diagnoses Using ICD-10-CM

Injuries, much like neoplasms and drugs, are given their own separate section in the ICD-10-CM index. Injuries are listed alphabetically by the source of the injury, with indented subcategories for more precise descriptions. For example, if a patient's injury was caused when they were hit by a thrown baseball during a game they were participating in, the indexed location would be "struck," then "object, thrown," in "sports, ball," and finally "baseball." As with disease codes, it is always considered best practice to go to the code location in the tabular list to verify before reporting, because some codes may require an additional character or characters that are not listed in the index.

Coding Drug-Related Diagnoses Using ICD-10-CM

Like neoplasms and injuries, diagnoses involving drugs have a special section in the ICD-10-CM index. The table of drugs and chemicals provides an alphabetical list for all common drugs and chemicals found in medical diagnoses, with subcategories for more precise definitions. For example, if a patient was exposed to ammonia fumes from a household cleaner, it would be listed under **"ammonia (fumes) (gas) (vapor),"** then **"liquid (household)."** The table also provides six categories for how the substance was used, as follows:

- **Poisoning, accidental**, when a patient unintentionally consumed toxic amounts of a substance
- **Poisoning, intentional, self-harm**, when a patient intentionally consumed toxic amounts of a substance
- **Poisoning, assault**, when a patient was exposed to toxic amounts of a substance by another individual
- **Poisoning, undetermined**, for when the cause of the patient's poisoning is unclear or unlisted
- **Adverse effect**, when a patient has a poor response (such as an allergic response) to a drug or substance
- **Underdosing**, when a patient is given an insufficient amount of a drug

Most codes will be found in the "T" section of ICD-10-CM. Always check the code in the tabular list before reporting it.

Chapter Quiz

Ready to see how well you retained what you just read? Scan the QR code to go directly to the chapter quiz interface for this study guide. If you're using a computer, simply visit the bonus page at **mometrix.com/bonus948/cpc** and click the Chapter Quizzes link.

Healthcare Common Procedure Coding System (HCPCS) Level II

Transform passive reading into active learning! After immersing yourself in this chapter, put your comprehension to the test by taking a quiz. The insights you gained will stay with you longer this way. Scan the QR code to go directly to the chapter quiz interface for this study guide. If you're using a computer, simply visit the bonus page at **mometrix.com/bonus948/cpc** and click the Chapter Quizzes link.

Modifiers

Coding System (HCPCS) Modifiers

Modifiers are alphabetic, numeric, or alphanumeric codes that are added to the end of CPT and HCPCS Level II codes to report specific modifications or alterations to the service or medical equipment without altering the code itself. These modifiers are used to more accurately report the procedure that the code describes for the purposes of billing and reimbursement of providers and suppliers.

When multiple modifiers may be appended to a single code, they must be listed in a specific way to be accurate. **Functional** modifiers, which alter the actual pricing of a procedure, are reported first in sequence. **Informational** modifiers, which clarify certain aspects of a procedure, such as laterality or anatomical position, are reported after functional modifiers. For example, if a bilateral procedure (modifier 50, an informational modifier) is discontinued (modifier 53, a functional modifier), then the ordering of the codes would be (CPT procedure code)-53-50.

Common HCPCS Modifiers Used with CPT Codes

Although HCPCS provides a wide variety of modifiers to cover different situations, not every modifier will be used regularly while coding procedures. Some modifiers are more common than others, and it pays to keep them in mind. These modifiers include the following:

22	Increased procedural service, meaning that the service was greater than what is typically required
26	Indicates the professional component, meaning that the individual who performs the procedure uses equipment or staff provided by a separate facility
51	Multiple procedures performed during a single session
52	Reduced services, meaning the service was less than what is typically required
53	Discontinued procedure, meaning the service was stopped due to circumstances
59	Distinct services, to indicate a procedure that is distinctly separate from other procedures performed in the same session
76	Repeat service by the same physician or other qualified healthcare professional

HCPCS Modifiers for Anatomic Positioning with CPT Codes

Certain HCPCS modifiers are used to indicate where on the body a procedure is performed. Generally speaking, some codes are required to determine the **laterality** of a procedure, such as the following:

50	Bilateral (both sides) procedure
LT	A procedure done on the left side
RT	A procedure done on the right side

Other codes are used to define a **specific location**, typically used for the eyelids, fingers, toes, and arteries, such as the following:

- **E1 and E2**: Upper and lower left side of the eyelid
- **E3 and E4**: Upper and lower right side of the eyelid
- **FA, F1, F2, F3, and F4**: Thumb through fifth digit, left hand
- **F5, F6, F7, F8, and F9**: Thumb through fifth digit, right hand
- **TA, T1, T2, T3, and T4**: Great toe through fifth digit, left foot
- **T5, T6, T7, T8, and T9**: Great toe through fifth digit, right foot
- **LC, LD, and LM**: The left circumflex, left anterior descending, and left main coronary arteries
- **RC and RI**: The right coronary and ramus intermedius coronary artery

Take note in the code descriptions of which of these modifiers are not used with that particular code.

HCPCS Modifiers for Payable Services Within a Global Package

Certain HCPCS modifiers are used during surgeries that are considered to be within what CPT refers to as a global package. A global package, as defined by CPT, consists of all procedures that occur before, during, and after (within a certain period of time) a specific surgical procedure, including any complications or postsurgical pain management. The modifiers commonly used for these include the following:

24	Unrelated E/M services by the same physician during the postoperative period
25	Significant, separate E/M service by the same physician on the same day as the procedure
57	The decision for surgery is made, such as in an emergency situation
58	Staged (i.e., done in stages over time) procedures by the same physician during the postoperative period
78	Unplanned return to the operating room by the same physician following the initial or a related procedure during the postoperative period
79	Unrelated procedure or service provided by the same physician during the postoperative period

Supplies

General Rules for Coding

HCPCS supply codes are five-character alphanumeric codes used when coding medical supplies and services provided via Medicare and other similar insurance providers. HCPCS codes are differentiated from CPT codes in that they begin with a letter as opposed to a number, although they share a similar reporting method. Whenever a specific drug or device is mentioned in a procedure code and is noted as being provided to a patient with Medicare, an HCPCS code should be used. When coding from HCPCS, first check the alphabetical index in order to locate the appropriate code, and then check in the appropriate section to confirm the code selection before adding it.

Locations and Categorizations of Supply Codes

Medical supply codes—meaning physical, nondrug equipment and supplies used in the treating of patients—are spread throughout HCPCS in a variety of categories. Generally speaking, medical supplies are divided into the following locations:

- **A4206 through A8004**: Medical and surgical supplies, such as gauze, scalpels, and drainage tubes
- **B4034 through B9999:** Enteral and parenteral therapy supplies
- **C1713 through C9899**: Outpatient prospective payment system, including implantable equipment such as pacemakers
- **E0100 through E8002:** Durable medical equipment, such as wheelchairs or commode chairs
- **K0001 through K0900**: Temporary durable medical equipment codes
- **L5000 through L9900**: Prosthetics and implants, such as extremity replacements and hernia mesh

Codes in these sections are organized alphabetically by the **general category** of equipment, followed by the **specific type of equipment.**

Medications

Coding of Drugs and Medications

The majority of drugs and medications are listed in section "J" of the HCPCS Level II codebook. These codes cover drugs that are administered via methods other than oral consumption, such as injection or inhalation, and they include a wide variety of pharmaceuticals. Certain other drugs, such as chemotherapy medications and oral medicines, can be found in section "Q" of HCPCS. Codes in section "J" are organized initially by the **method of administration** (such as injection), then alphabetically by the **name of the drug**, and then by dosage. Some drugs will have additional, alternative names listed underneath the description (e.g., the drug baclofen may also be referred to as Gablofen or Lioresal). Always read the procedure notes to confirm the name of the drug that is administered.

Effectively Coding Drugs and Biologicals Using Appendix A

HCPCS provides a table of drugs and biological agents, generic and brand name, in **Appendix A** of the HCPCS book. In addition to an alphabetical list, the index includes the standard unit of measurement, the route of application, and the appropriate code to be used for each drug. The unit of measurement determines how many times the code is used based on the amount given. For example, if a patient is given 50 mg of acetaminophen, that would be five units because acetaminophen is described in doses of 10 mg. This table should be used in tandem with the index in order to accurately report drugs listed in the procedure notes provided.

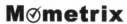

Professional Services

Service codes, meaning services that are performed on or with a patient for the purposes of treatment or investigation, are spread throughout HCPCS in a variety of categories. Generally speaking, professional services are divided into the following locations:

- **A0021 through A0999**: Transportation services, including ambulances
- **A9150 through A9999**: Administrative, investigational, and miscellaneous diagnostic services
- **G0008 through G9987**: Professional services and procedures such as oncology
- **H0001 through H2037**: Alcohol and drug abuse treatment
- **L0112 through L4631**: Orthotic procedures and services
- **M0075 through M0301**: Medical services not otherwise classified
- **P2028 through P9615**: Pathology and laboratory services
- **R0070 through R0076**: Diagnostic radiology services
- **V2020 through V2799**: Vision services
- **V5008 through V5364**: Hearing services

Codes of these types are organized by the **specific services** that are involved.

Chapter Quiz

Ready to see how well you retained what you just read? Scan the QR code to go directly to the chapter quiz interface for this study guide. If you're using a computer, simply visit the bonus page at **mometrix.com/bonus948/cpc** and click the Chapter Quizzes link.

Coding Guidelines

Transform passive reading into active learning! After immersing yourself in this chapter, put your comprehension to the test by taking a quiz. The insights you gained will stay with you longer this way. Scan the QR code to go directly to the chapter quiz interface for this study guide. If you're using a computer, simply visit the bonus page at **mometrix.com/bonus948/cpc** and click the Chapter Quizzes link.

ICD-10-CM Official Guidelines

Common Coding Conventions

The ICD-10-CM guidebook uses a variety of terms, abbreviations, and symbols to quickly and accurately provide information with minimal space requirements. Knowledge of these conventions is necessary to quickly code diagnoses. Common coding conventions used by the ICD-10-CM guidebook include items from the following table:

Item		Use
-	Hyphen	Used in the index to indicate that there are additional characters associated with the code.
NEC	Not elsewhere classified	This means there isn't a code for that specific condition.
NOS	Not otherwise specified	Shorthand for "unspecified."
[]	Brackets	Used for manifestation codes in the index and synonyms or explanatory phrases in the tabular list.
()	Parentheses	Enclose supplementary words or terms used for the condition.
INCLUDES		The conditions listed after this are covered by this code.
EXCLUDES1		The conditions listed after this are never reported with this code.
EXCLUDES2		The conditions listed after this may be reported with this code.
Code First		Indicates a code or type of code that should be sequenced before this code.

General Guidelines

When coding using ICD-10-CM, there are general guidelines that should always be followed in order to accurately and correctly report diagnoses. As a general rule, the following general guidelines should be followed when reporting ICD-10-CM codes:

- **In an outpatient setting, only code confirmed conditions or diseases.** If a condition is only suspected or possible but not confirmed, then it should not be coded. In an inpatient setting, a diagnosis that is suspected or possible may be reported if a definitive diagnosis has not been documented at the time of discharge.
- **Code to the highest level of specificity.** Do not simply select a general code if a more focused and precise code is otherwise available.
- **Codes provided should support the medical necessity of treatment.** The codes provided must accurately reflect the available facts. In other words, no speculation is allowed.
- Each unique code should be reported only once per encounter.
- Codes should be sequenced in the order of what is most responsible for the patient encounter.

Coding Signs and Symptoms

Signs and symptoms refer to non-diagnosis codes used for identifying individual, unrelated conditions, such as sneezing or fever. Such issues may or may not be associated with other conditions listed in the procedural notes. ICD-10-CM has a few guidelines related to this particular case of coding:

- If signs and symptoms **are present and a definitive diagnosis has not been confirmed**, then any listed signs and symptoms should be coded individually using the appropriate codes found in the tabular index.
- If the signs and symptoms are an integral part of—or are routinely associated with—the confirmed diagnosis, then they are not separately coded.
- If the signs and symptoms **are not routinely associated with the confirmed diagnosis,** then they should be coded individually with the appropriate codes.

Coding Sequelae

Sequela (plural "sequelae") is a medical term used for leftover or residual conditions, typically caused by the initial problem, that occur after an illness or injury has been handled. Examples of sequelae include things like chronic arthritis after fracturing a wrist, severe scarring after a burn, or aphasia after a brain hemorrhage. Sequelae may occur immediately following the condition, or they may occur months or even years later; there is no time limit for a sequela to occur. When a sequela is diagnosed in a patient, the **sequela condition** is coded first, followed by the illness or injury responsible for the current condition. For example, if a patient develops an intellectual disability due to poliomyelitis, the codes sequenced should be F79 (unspecified intellectual disability), followed by B91 (sequela of poliomyelitis). The exception to this is if the code identifies the condition as following another condition, such as I69.120 (aphasia following nontraumatic intracerebral hemorrhage).

Coding HIV

The ICD-10-CM guidelines specify how to appropriately code patients who have human immunodeficiency virus (HIV) and how it interacts with related conditions, as outlined below:

- Only code confirmed cases of HIV. In addition, the code for HIV (B20) should be included in all future cases of a patient with confirmed HIV.
- If a patient's condition is **related to HIV**, then the first diagnosis should be HIV (code B20), followed by the related conditions.
- If an HIV-positive patient is admitted for an **unrelated condition**, code the unrelated condition first, and then code the HIV.
- If a patient has **inconclusive or asymptomatic HIV status**, code B20 first if the condition is HIV related, or code the condition first followed by code Z21 if the condition isn't HIV related.

Sequencing Neoplasm Codes

Neoplasm codes are mostly located in their specific section of the index in ICD-10-CM, and they have several guidelines for the proper sequencing of multiple types of codes. Common sequencing codes are as follows:

- When coding treatment of a **primary malignancy**, code the primary site first and then any secondary metastasized sites.
- When coding treatment of **secondary malignancy**, code the metastatic sites first and then the primary site.

- If the patient is undergoing treatment for a **complication** related to a neoplasm, code the complication first and then the neoplasm.
- If a patient is being treated for **anemia related to a neoplasm**, code the neoplasm first and then code D63.0 (anemia in neoplastic disease).
- If a patient is being seen for a **pathological fracture due to a neoplasm**, code the focus of the treatment first.
- If a primary malignancy has been excised but **further treatment** is being performed, code the primary malignancy until treatment is completed. Afterward, if there is no evidence of malignancy at that site, use the appropriate code from category Z85.

Coding Diabetes

ICD-10-CM has several guidelines for properly coding diabetes mellitus, one of the most common endocrine diseases. Common guidelines are as follows:

- If the type of diabetes mellitus is not specified in the procedure notes or the medical record, code the condition as type 2 diabetes mellitus (E11).
- If the type of diabetes mellitus is not specified and the procedure notes include the use of insulin, code type 2 diabetes mellitus and include an additional code from category Z79 to identify long-term use of insulin or hypoglycemic drugs.
- If the type of diabetes is gestational diabetes caused by pregnancy, assign a code from subcategory O24.4 instead of the standard diabetes code.

Coding Hypertensive Heart Disease and Chronic Kidney Disease

Hypertensive heart disease and chronic kidney disease are two conditions that are commonly **comorbid** (meaning they occur simultaneously) in a patient, enough that the situation has dedicated guidelines when it is coded in ICD-10-CM. Unless the procedural notes state that the two conditions are unrelated, the condition should be sequenced as follows:

1. Code from combination category **I13** for hypertension with heart and kidney involvement.
2. If heart failure is present, use the appropriate code from category **I50.**
3. Code from category **N18** to identify the stage of chronic kidney disease.
4. If the patient is suffering from acute renal failure as well, code the level of renal failure last in the sequence.

Coding External Causes of Morbidity

External causes of morbidity is the term that ICD-10-CM uses to indicate an injury or condition that was caused by outside forces, such as car accidents, falls, natural disasters, and so on. These codes can be used to elaborate on how a condition was caused; the intent behind it (accidental, intentional, or otherwise); where the event that caused the condition occurred; as well as the patient's status, whether military, civilian, etc.

External-cause codes are not sequenced first, and they are only used in conjunction with codes from other ranges if an external cause is mentioned. Typically, they'll be used with injuries or poisonings. When coding, use as many external cause codes as necessary to fully represent the condition as it is explained in the procedural notes.

Coding Patient Histories

Patient histories are coded using codes from section "Z" in the tabular list, covering code categories **Z80 through Z87.89, Z91.4 through Z91.52, and Z92.** History codes are divided into two different types: **personal** and **family.** Personal history codes are used when a procedure mentions a patient's past medical condition that may be relevant to the current condition or requires monitoring, and they are used in conjunction with follow-up codes. Family history codes are used when the procedural notes mention that a patient has familial history that may put them at risk for certain conditions, and they are used in conjunction with screening codes to establish medical necessity. Either type is acceptable on a medical record for the reason for the visit.

Screening Codes

Screening codes are used for encounters that focus on testing for signs and precursors of diseases in seemingly healthy individuals, typically for the purposes of early detection and treatment of a condition. Screening codes are listed in section "Z" of the tabular list in sections **"Z11"** through **"Z13"** and "**Z36**," and they are used to indicate that a screening has been planned. If the purpose of the encounter is specifically for the screening exam, then the screening code is sequenced first. If a condition is discovered during the screening, the code for the condition should be sequenced separately after the screening code.

CPT

Common Conventions for Codes

The CPT guidebook uses a variety of symbols and formatting in order to present information in a way that can be easily referenced and understood by the reader. Knowledge of these conventions helps the reader to quickly understand codes at a glance and how they are referenced. Important conventions for coding are listed below:

- **Indentation**: A code description that is indented is used to indicate a modification of the non-indented code listed above it. For example, the code 21462, "with interdental fixation," is indented underneath code 21461, "open treatment of mandibular fracture; without interdental fixation." Therefore, the appropriate way to read code 21462 is "open treatment of mandibular fracture; with interdental fixation."
- **+**: The "plus" sign indicates that the code is an **add-on code**, meaning that it adds on to an existing code. Add-on codes cannot be reported on their own.
- **⊘**: The "no" symbol indicates that the code is exempted from modifier 51.
- **Red text**: Bright red text indicates that the code in question has been moved to another location in the CPT guidebook. Read the text to see where the code has been moved to.

Criteria Used for Code Categories

CPT codes are defined by the American Medical Association and are separated into three categories based on the frequency of clinical use, clearance by the appropriate oversight bodies, and levels of monetary value. CPT code categories are listed below:

- **Category I**: This category is used for procedures cleared or approved by the FDA that are frequently performed and documented. These codes make up the bulk of CPT's codes and cover E/M, anesthesia, surgery, radiology, pathology, and laboratory and medicine. These codes have five digits.
- **Category II**: This category is used for reporting procedures that are usually included in E/M or clinical services but are not associated with the typical fees or values. These codes are made up of four numbers followed by the letter F.
- **Category III**: This category covers codes used for temporary or experimental procedures or services. Codes in this category are made up of four numbers followed by the letter T.

Reporting of Unlisted Procedures

Despite its regular updates, the CPT codebook does not list every single procedure that may be performed by a physician or other qualified healthcare provider. If a procedure is performed that is currently unlisted by CPT, each section of CPT has a designated code, typically ending in 99, that is used to report unlisted procedures or services. For example, an unlisted procedure involving the lacrimal system would use code 68899. These codes should only be used if a more appropriate code is not available or if CPT references the unlisted procedure code's use in a parenthetical note.

Parentheticals

Parentheticals, also known as parenthetical notes, refer to additional information used to supplement a procedural code or to aid in accurately coding procedures in CPT. Parentheticals are so named for the use of parentheses to bracket either end of the note. Parentheticals are used in several different ways, including presenting additional codes that may be involved in a procedure, listing codes that should or should not be reported in conjunction with a particular code, guiding the reader to related procedures, and other advisory notes. When in doubt on a procedure, always check for any parenthetical notes that may be included.

HCPCS

Common Symbols and Conventions

HCPCS uses symbols and text conventions to provide necessary information to code Medicare procedures without taking up excess space. Knowledge of these symbols and conventions will allow a coder to quickly and accurately code procedures in HCPCS. Commonly used conventions are listed below:

- **Letter in a block**: A letter in a blue block is used to identify circumstances affecting payment: **C** means carrier judgment, **D** means that special coverage instructions apply, **I** means not payable by Medicare, **M** means noncovered by Medicare, and **S** means noncovered by Medicare statute.
- **Colored text**: Colored text is used for indicators: **Green** is used for ambulatory surgical center (ASC) indicators, **red** is used for ambulatory payment calculator indicators, and **purple** indicates an ASC-approved procedure.
- **Blue text**: Blue text is used for alerts, such as "Service not separately priced by Part B."
- **DME**: This text in a purple box means that the procedure is paid under a durable medical equipment fee schedule.
- **MIPS**: This text in a light-blue box indicates that the code is covered under the merit-based incentive payment system (MIPS).

Types of Codes

HCPCS covers a variety of codes that are classified as Level II codes, comparable to CPT's Level I codes. The HCPCS is used to efficiently code and process claims for products and services across a wide variety of fields and states, including a wide variety of manufacturers. Most of the codes in HCPCS can be divided into the three categories listed below:

- **Permanent national codes**: Permanent national codes are maintained by the Centers for Medicare and Medicare Services (CMS) and are used by all public and private health insurers. These codes make up the bulk of the HCPCS codes provided.
- **Miscellaneous codes**: These codes are used when a supplier or provider submits a bill for a service or item that currently lacks an appropriate permanent national code. These codes are typically used for items or services that are rarely used.

- **Temporary national codes**: Temporary national codes are used to meet the operational needs of a particular insurer within a short time frame. Unlike miscellaneous codes, temporary national codes may be made into permanent codes.

Chapter Quiz

Ready to see how well you retained what you just read? Scan the QR code to go directly to the chapter quiz interface for this study guide. If you're using a computer, simply visit the bonus page at **mometrix.com/bonus948/cpc** and click the Chapter Quizzes link.

Compliance and Regulatory

Transform passive reading into active learning! After immersing yourself in this chapter, put your comprehension to the test by taking a quiz. The insights you gained will stay with you longer this way. Scan the QR code to go directly to the chapter quiz interface for this study guide. If you're using a computer, simply visit the bonus page at **mometrix.com/bonus948/cpc** and click the Chapter Quizzes link.

Medicare

Medicare Part A

Medicare Part A is part of the United States government's insurance plan that insures inpatient hospital care and visits for the beneficiary. Medicare Part A covers hospital stays, room and food, medical tests, doctors' fees, skilled nursing care, hospice care, and some forms of home healthcare. Individuals are allowed to enroll on their 65th birthday, and if the individual pays into the Supplemental Security Income system for 10 years, it does not require a monthly premium. A patient may still pay some copays depending on the services required. Coverage is based on national coverage decisions as well as local decisions made by companies in each state on what is considered medically necessary.

Medicare Part B

Medicare Part B is part of the United States government's insurance plan that insures outpatient care, including doctors' visits, routine physicals and wellness checks, mammograms, x-rays, laboratory work, home health, physical and occupational therapy, infusion clinics, diabetes, prostate screenings, and other medically necessary and preventative services. This also includes ambulance services and durable medical equipment. Premiums must be paid, but they may be deducted from an individual's Supplemental Security Income check, as well as deductibles and copays if a service is not covered. Coverage is based on national coverage decisions as well as local decisions made by companies in each state on what is considered medically necessary.

Medicare Part C

Medicare Part C, also known as Medicare Advantage, is part of the United States government's insurance plan that is administered by private insurance companies that are contracted with Medicare. Medicare Part C combines elements of parts A, B, and D, and it covers health and wellness plans, vision, hearing, dental, medications, and some hospital and doctor visits. Part C typically involves a health maintenance organization, a preferred provider organization, or other similar insurance company, and a beneficiary must pay copays, premiums, and deductibles for services rendered. Typically, the patient will select a care provider from the providing company's network of physicians and professionals. An individual can enroll in Medicare Part C at age 65 or during open enrollment.

Medicare Part D

Medicare Part D is part of the United States government's insurance plan that assists in supporting prescription drug coverage. Medicare Part D is considered optional, but it is available to all Medicare beneficiaries who are willing to pay the fees. Coverage for Medicare Part D is provided by private companies and can be purchased by itself or can be used to supplement other plans, including Medicare Part C. Patients must pay premiums, copays, and deductibles for the plan, and they must select from pharmacies within the provider's established network. An individual can enroll in Medicare Part D at age 65 or during open enrollment.

CODING

PAYMENT POLICY

TYPES OF PAYERS THAT CODERS BILL

The purpose of medical coders is to code diagnoses and services in order to effectively bill health insurance for the costs of services. Whereas some patients pay for their medical expenses out of pocket with their own money, most patients will have one or more health plans that are billed. Most of these payers fall under three categories:

- **Commercial carriers** are private insurance companies that offer medical insurance for groups and individuals. They include organizations such as Blue Cross/Blue Shield, Aetna, and other major providers. Contracts provided by these companies cover a wide variety of services and individual plans.
- **Medicare** is the United States' primary government-funded insurance, paid for by the federal government and administered by CMS. Medicare is available to individuals older than age 65 and those who are blind, disabled, or suffering from permanent kidney failure or ESRD. Medicare is made up of multiple parts (Medicare Parts A, B, C, and D).
- **Medicaid** is an insurance assistance program sponsored at the federal and state level for low-income individuals, especially pregnant women and children. Medicaid coverage varies from state to state, but it must adhere to certain federal guidelines.

MIPS

The merit-based incentive payment system (MIPS) is one of two programs used to determine Medicare payments in order to promote improvement and innovation in clinical activities. Established in April 2015 as part of the Medicare Access and Children's Health Insurance Program Reauthorization Act, MIPS measures the performance of participating providers (referred to as eligible clinicians) based on the **quality** of performance, **promoting interoperability** by using electronic health record technology, **improvement activities** such as care coordination and patient safety, and **cost** of care. The combined aggregate score determines whether participating eligible clinicians receive an adjustment (positive, negative, or neutral) to their Medicare reimbursement.

APMS

Alternative payment models (APMs) are one of two tracks used to determine Medicare payments for services rendered. Established in April 2015 as part of the Medicare Access and Children's Health Insurance Program Reauthorization Act, APMs are meant to ensure that patients, especially patients suffering from chronic conditions, receive care while avoiding unnecessary errors or duplication of services. Over time, providers who receive a substantial percentage of their Medicare Part B payments or see a substantial percentage of their Medicare patients through an APM can earn a 5% yearly incentive payment. Unlike with MIPS, there are a wide variety of APMs available, depending on the specialty and provider type.

PLACE OF SERVICE REPORTING

PLACE OF SERVICE CODES

A place of service code is a two-digit code used on a healthcare professional's service claim document to show what setting the professional's services were provided in. The place of service code list is maintained by CMS, and it can greatly affect the reimbursement rate of the professional depending on the code used when billing Medicare, Medicaid, or private insurance. Place of service codes are divided into categories based on whether treatment takes place in a medical facility or not. Place of service codes are separate from codes used for diagnosis and procedure identification, and they are not coded alongside them.

Facility vs. Non-Facility Place of Service Codes

Place of service codes are divided into facility and non-facility codes. Facility codes cover services provided by hospitals, skilled nursing facilities, or ambulatory surgical centers. Non-facility codes cover all other locations.

Facility Codes	Non-facility Codes
02: Telehealth **21**: Inpatient hospital **22**: On-campus outpatient hospital **23**: Emergency room (hospital) **24**: Ambulatory surgical center **26**: Military treatment facility **31**: Skilled nursing facility **34**: Hospice **41**: Ambulance (land) **42**: Ambulance (air/water) **51**: Inpatient psychiatric facility **52**: Psychiatric facility (partial hospitalization) **53**: Community mental health center **56**: Residential psychiatric treatment center **61**: Comprehensive inpatient rehabilitation facility	**01**: Pharmacy **03**: School **04**: Homeless shelter **09**: Prison/correctional facility **11**: Office **12**: Home **13**: Assisted-living facility **14**: Group home **15**: Mobile unit **16**: Temporary lodging **17**: Walk-in retail health clinic **20**: Urgent care facility **25**: Birthing center **32**: Nursing facility **33**: Custodial care facility **49**: Independent clinic **50**: Federally qualified health center **54**: Intermediate care facility for individuals with intellectual disabilities **55**: Residential substance abuse treatment facility **57**: Nonresidential substance abuse treatment facility **60**: Mass immunization center **62**: Comprehensive outpatient rehabilitation facility **65**: ESRD treatment facility **71**: State/local public health clinic **72**: Rural health clinic **81**: Independent laboratory **99**: Other place of service

Compliance and Regulatory

Fraud and Abuse

Fraud in Medical Coding

It is possible to commit fraud as a medical coder—fraud being the criminal deception of an individual or organization for financial gain. In this case, fraud involves intentionally overcharging insurance companies or falsely reporting services that were not provided. Common examples of coding fraud include the following:

- Applying a higher-paying billing code to a professional service, also known as upcoding
- Billing services provided or performed by nurses, residents, and staff under codes that are used only for a physician's duties
- Billing the components of a bundled code separately, also known as unbundling

- Billing a treatment that was performed during a single encounter as if it occurred over multiple days, also known as split billing
- Reporting a higher number of units of service than what was provided

Abuse in Medical Coding

While fraud is intentional behavior, abuse happens when a service is unknowingly overcharged or misused. Although abuse is not done deliberately, it is still illegal, and perpetrators will be subject to monetary penalties or incarceration. The best way to avoid this type of improper billing practice is to participate in self-audits and be fully aware of the compliance programs created by an organization or entity for which you are employed. Common examples of abuse include the following:

- Charging excessively for services or supplies
- Billing for services that were not medically necessary or, if they were medically necessary, not having the documentation to prove medical necessity
- Waiving a patient's deductible or out-of-pocket costs

Compliance Audits

Regular audits are typically performed to ensure accurate coding, maximize quality and reimbursement of services, and to ensure compliance with proper practices and standards and preventing coding fraud. Typically, compliance audits are performed by a certified outside party. Coding audits can be either **prospective** or **retrospective.** A prospective audit is performed before a claim is fully submitted in order to catch mistakes before they're made. Retrospective audits, conversely, are performed after claims are processed, and they can typically cover a percentage of claims submitted by an individual or service provider. Failing an audit can lead to disciplinary action, either for an individual coder or for a service provider.

OIG

Established in 1976, the Office of Inspector General (OIG) is a government agency tasked with maintaining the integrity of Health and Human Services programs. Typically, this means assisting the medical industry in overseeing Medicare and Medicaid guidelines, preventing fraud and abuse, ensuring compliance, educating the public, and taking action against service providers who fail to comply with their established standards. The OIG also performs audits and provides guidelines for compliance plans that are used by medical service providers. In the event of fraud or other criminal activities, the OIG has authority to exclude individuals or organizations from receiving payment from federal healthcare programs such as Medicare and Medicaid.

OIG Compliance Plan

An OIG compliance plan is an essential document that almost all healthcare providers and healthcare facilities use to ensure appropriate guidance and compliance with the OIG's guidelines and to minimize claim errors. Compliance plans, per the OIG's official recommendations, include seven key components, which are summarized as follows:

- Conducting internal monitoring and auditing, including performing periodic audits for the purpose of evaluation
- Developing and implementing clearly written compliance and practice standards
- Designating or contracting a compliance officer or officers to monitor compliance efforts and enforce standards
- Conducting appropriate training and education on the best practices and standards for procedures

- Responding appropriately to violations and taking steps to correct problems
- Developing and maintaining open lines of communication between staff and employees
- Enforcing disciplinary standards

National Correct Coding Initiative (NCCI) Edits

NCCI

The National Correct Coding Initiative (NCCI) is a program created by CMS to implement and promote correct coding methodologies and curtail improper coding at a national level. The NCCI's policies are based on current coding practices and conventions included in CPT, an analysis of standard medical practice, and local and national coverage determinations. Essentially, the NCCI helps to clarify codes that are used, decide which codes are bundled together or kept separate, and show effective dates and **procedure-to-procedure (PTP)** edits of CPT procedure codes with included rationales. It is updated quarterly.

Presentation of Information

The NCCI provides coders with a method to assess whether codes should be used together or not. When using the NCCI, the information is usually presented as follows:

Heading	Column 1	Column 2	* = In Existence Prior to 1996	Effective Date	Deletion Date * = No Data	Modifier 0 = Not allowed 1 = Allowed 9 = Non-applicable	PTP Edit Rationale
Example	11042	0213T		20100701	*	0	Misuse of column 2 code with column 1 code

- **Column 1**: The primary or major procedure or service performed.
- **Column 2**: The secondary or lesser service performed.
- **In Existence Prior to 1996**: This column indicates if the edit existed prior to 1996, when the NCCI became standard procedure.
- **Effective Date**: The date that the edit came into effect.
- **Deletion Date**: The date that the edit was deleted (if applicable).
- **Modifier**: This indicates whether a correct coding modifier allows a code pair in columns 1 and 2 to bypass the edit. A 0 indicates that the combination of codes should never, under any circumstance, be reported together; a 1 indicates that the combination of codes may be reported together with the use of a coding modifier; and a 9 indicates that the combination of codes is reportable on their own, and does not require the use of a coding modifier.
- **PTP Edit Rationale**: The rationale behind the PTP edit.

National Coverage Determination (NCD)

A national coverage determination (NCD) is a type of determination guideline for whether Medicare will pay for a particular item, service, or treatment. Determinations are made by CMS at the request of external parties (such as manufacturers or health plans) to determine whether the item or service can be used for a specific diagnosis based on **medical necessity** (e.g., if a procedure or item is considered appropriate for treatment). As the name suggests, NCDs are guidelines established at a national level, and all Medicare contractors are obligated to follow them. If the procedure is covered, then Medicare will reimburse the provider.

Local Coverage Determination (LCD)

A local coverage determination (LCD) is a type of determination guideline for whether Medicare will pay for a particular item, service, or treatment. Unlike an NCD, an LCD has jurisdiction only within a specific region. If an NCD does not exist for a particular item or service, or if an NCD requires additional definition, then it is up to a **Medicare administrative contractor (MAC)** to rule on whether or not that service or item can be reimbursed based on medical necessity, thus creating an LCD within that contractor's region. Lists of LCDs are published regularly in order to provide coders with appropriate guidance.

HIPAA

Created in 1996, the Health Insurance Portability and Accountability Act (HIPAA) is a federal law that establishes protections for sensitive health information, sets national standards for the security of electronic healthcare transactions, and institutes measures to prevent healthcare fraud and abuse. Most noticeably for medical coders, HIPAA defines privacy rules in regard to patient information and sets national standards for code sets and unique identifiers for health plans, health providers, and employers. HIPAA's privacy rules apply to all covered entities, including doctors' offices, clinics, psychologists, dentists, nursing homes, pharmacies, health insurance companies, and healthcare clearinghouses.

Privacy Guidelines

HIPAA stipulates that only the **minimum necessary** amount of a patient's medical and personal information should be shared or provided to satisfy a specific medical purpose, and only to those who require it. For example, a nurse working with an HIV-positive patient should not share that patient's HIV status with a peer while the nurse is off duty.

This standard does have some exceptions; information may be disclosed if:

- It is required to provide treatment.
- It is disclosed to the subject of the information.
- It is pursuant to an authorization of an individual.
- It is required for compliance with HIPAA's rules.
- It is disclosed to the Department of Health and Human Services for purposes of enforcement.
- It is required by other laws.

Advance Beneficiary Notices (ABNs)

An advance beneficiary notice (ABN) is a standardized, one-page Medicare form used to notify a patient that a procedure, treatment, or service may not be covered by Medicare. An ABN explains why Medicare may deny the procedure or procedures, and it is used to protect the provider's financial interests by creating a paper trail if Medicare denies reimbursement. An ABN alone is not sufficient; the patient should also be provided with a specific explanation as to why a service may be denied. An ABN also cannot be used to bill a patient for additional fees beyond what Medicare reimburses. ABNs may not be used for emergency or urgent care situations.

Relative Value Units (RVUs)

Relative value units (RVUs) are a measure of value established for Medicare as part of the **resource-based relative value scale (RBRVS)**. The intention was to create a stable and nonvariable rate for Medicare payments for physician services, rather than the more inconsistent system that existed before. RVUs themselves have no financial value; instead, they inform how much a particular service is worth (for example, a service with an RVU of 3 is worth three times as much as a service with an RVU of 1). RVUs cover three different factors: the **physician's work**, which represents the time, skill, and difficulty of the service provided; the **practice expense**, which reflects the costs of personnel, supplies, and overhead; and the **liability/malpractice expense** for the purposes of insurance.

Calculation

The RBRVS is a formula that is used to calculate how much Medicare reimburses a provider for procedures. CMS annually publishes this information on its website and provides comprehensive listings for all RVUs. The formula used for calculating reimbursement is as follows:

$$[(\text{W RVU} \times \text{W GPCI}) + (\text{PE RVU} \times \text{PE GPCI}) + (\text{MP RVU} \times \text{MP GPCI})] \times \text{conversion factor}$$

- **RVU**: the relative value unit for work performed (W), physician's expense ([PE] facility or non-facility), and malpractice liability (MP)
- **GPCI**: the **geographic practice cost index**, which varies based on the location of the practice
- **Conversion factor:** a fixed dollar amount used to translate the resulting formula into fees

Chapter Quiz

Ready to see how well you retained what you just read? Scan the QR code to go directly to the chapter quiz interface for this study guide. If you're using a computer, simply visit the bonus page at mometrix.com/bonus948/cpc and click the Chapter Quizzes link.

CPC Practice Test #1

Want to take this practice test in an online interactive format?
Check out the bonus page, which includes interactive practice questions and much more: **mometrix.com/bonus948/cpc**

1. What is the correct code assignment for the percutaneous radiofrequency ablation of two liver tumors?

a. 47383
b. 47380
c. 47370
d. 47382

2. According to the OIG-issued General Compliance Program Guidance effective November 2023, what should be included in the compliance committee charter for a small entity?

a. A statement of meeting frequency
b. Discussion of provider salaries
c. Compliance assessment of the clinical nursing staff
d. A mandate for a formal disclosure program

3. Consultation codes are used to report a consultation to recommend care or treatment of a specific condition or problem if the consultation is initiated by which of the following people?

a. The patient
b. The mother of a minor
c. The caretaker
d. A social worker

4. What is the correct code assignment for mass spectrometry with chromatography drug screening?

a. 80305
b. 80307
c. 80306
d. 80320

5. What is the correct code assignment for a percutaneous transcatheter closure with implant of a congenital atrial-septal defect?

a. 33641
b. 93580
c. 33675
d. 93581

6. What is the correct code assignment for a first-stage partial transurethral resection of the prostate?

a. 52500
b. 52630
c. 52601
d. 52648

7. What is the ileum?

a. The uppermost, largest portion of the pelvic girdle
b. The posterior portion of the pelvic girdle
c. A slightly curved, triangular-shaped bone
d. The third part of the small intestine

8. Assign the correct diagnosis and procedure codes for the following encounter.

The patient presented with a nonhealing lesion over the scalp, which he has had for more than 5 years. He states that it has been growing slowly. Today, it measures 3 cm × 2.5 cm. The decision was made to excise the basal cell carcinoma lesion of the scalp. Surgery was scheduled, and preop instructions were given.

Procedure Note: The patient was placed in the supine position, and laryngeal mask anesthesia was carried out. Initially, the left arm was prepped with SoluPrep and isolated with drapes. A split-thickness skin graft was harvested from the left upper arm. The donor site was dressed with Acticoat. The lesion to be excised was marked out by a spherical outline with 1 cm clearance. The 4-cm diameter lesion was then excised. It was marked by a black stitch anteriorly and a blue stitch right laterally. Hemostasis was controlled. The harvested skin graft was placed on the recipient site and anchored with 4-0 sutures as well as staples. A tie-over dressing was used to stabilize the graft. The swab and instrument count was correct at the end of the procedure. The patient was transferred to the recovery room in stable condition. The pathology report confirms basal cell carcinoma of the scalp.

a. C44.41, 15100, 11624-51
b. C44.91, 11624, 15100-51
c. 15110, 11624-51, C44.91
d. 11624, 15110-51, C44.41

9. What is the correct code assignment for repair of transposition of the great arteries, Senning-type atrial baffle procedure, with cardiopulmonary bypass and closure of a ventricular septal defect?

a. 33771
b. 33780
c. 33770
d. 33776

10. The patient requires a full-length surgical stocking for the right leg. Assign the correct HCPCS Level II code.

a. A6536
b. A4495
c. A6537
d. A4510

CPC Practice Test

11. A patient presents to the office for follow-up for an acute episode of COVID-19 that required hospitalization. It is determined that the condition is resolved. The patient is counseled regarding symptoms of long COVID. Assign the correct ICD-10-CM codes.

a. Z86.19, Z09
b. Z09, Z86.16
c. Z86.16, Z09
d. Z09, U09.9

12. An elderly patient presents to primary care with a complaint of chronic arthritis due to a traumatic left hip fracture. Assign the correct ICD-10-CM code.

a. M19.90
b. M16.52
c. M12.552
d. M16.7

13. Assign the correct diagnosis and procedure codes for the following encounter.

A 64-year-old established female patient presents to the office for a follow-up for diet-controlled type 2 diabetes mellitus, which was diagnosed earlier this year, and hypertension. Blood sugars have been in the normal range since her last visit. Home blood pressures are good. 120/72 today in the office. She will continue the current dose of Aldactone. The patient remains overweight at 180 lb with a BMI of 35.15. She continues to go to yoga three times a week and walks for exercise on the weekend. She has lost an additional 6 pounds since her last weigh-in for a total of 24 pounds in 5 months. We discussed healthy eating habits, and we celebrated her continued success with dieting. She is to schedule another follow-up appointment for 3 months from now and will contact the office if any concerns arise in the interim. The total time spent for this visit was 21 minutes.

a. E11.9, I10, E66.3, Z68.35, 99213
b. E11.9, I10, E66.08, 99214
c. I10, E11.9, E66.3, Z68.35, 99214
d. E11.9, I10, E66.09, 99213

14. What is the correct code assignment for a bone density study, with dual-photon absorptiometry, of 1 or more sites?

a. 78350
b. 78351
c. 77081
d. 77080

15. A 39-year-old patient who is 2 days postpartum develops preeclampsia with hemolysis, elevated liver enzymes, and a low platelet count. Assign the correct ICD-10-CM code.

a. O14.25
b. O14.95
c. O14.15
d. O14.05

16. What is the correct code assignment for a right arthroscopic rotator cuff repair and a right distal shoulder claviculectomy during the same surgical setting?

a. 29824-RT, 29827-51-RT
b. 29827-RT, 29824-51-RT
c. 29824-RT, 29824-59-RT
d. 29827-RT, 29824-59-RT

17. Assign the correct diagnosis and procedure codes for the following encounter.

The patient presented to the emergency department with severe right flank pain and a temperature of 100.2 °F. A noncontrast abdominal CT scan revealed a 7-mm calculus in the proximal left ureter with hydronephrosis. The emergency department physician concurred with the radiological diagnosis. The patient was prescribed a narcotic pain medication and discharged to pass the stone naturally. An appropriate history and physical were performed, with medical decision-making of moderate complexity.

a. N20.1, N13.6, 74150, 99284
b. N13.2, 74150, 99284
c. N13.6, 74160, 99284
d. N13.2, R50.9, 74160, 99284

18. A patient undergoes percutaneous removal and replacement of an internally dwelling ureteral stent, with ultrasonic visualization. Assign the correct code for this procedure.

a. 50384
b. 50382
c. 50386
d. 50385

19. What is the correct code assignment for a secondary rhinoplasty with a major revision?

a. 30420
b. 30450
c. 30460
d. 30410

20. What category of ICD-10-CM diagnosis codes has sequencing priority over the other code categories?

a. COVID-19
b. Obstetrics
c. Human immunodeficiency virus (HIV) infections
d. Malignant neoplasms

21. What is the correct code assignment for a flexible bronchoscopy with fluoroscopic guidance and tracheal dilation with placement of tracheal stents?

a. 31636
b. 31631
c. 31638
d. 31630

22. What is the correct code assignment for extracapsular phacoemulsification cataract removal of the left eye with endoscopic cyclophotocoagulation?

a. 66988-LT
b. 66982-LT
c. 66987-LT
d. 66984-LT

23. A patient presents to urgent care for possible fracture of the right index finger. An x-ray is performed and is negative. It is determined that the finger should be supported with a prefabricated finger splint. Assign the correct HCPCS Level II code.

a. S8450-F6
b. Q4049-F6
c. A4570-RT
d. S8450-F1

24. What is the correct code assignment for a colonoscopy with directed submucosal saline injection of a lesion for endoscopic mucosal resection?

a. 45381
b. 45381, 45390-51
c. 45390, 45381-51
d. 45390

25. What is the correct anesthesia code assignment for radical mastectomy of the left breast?

a. 00402
b. 00404
c. 00406
d. 00400

26. What is the correct code assignment for a work-related disability examination with completion of reports performed by other than the treating physician?

a. 99450
b. 99455
c. 99456
d. 99242

27. What is the correct code assignment for the excision of a 275 g uterus via a laparoscopic-assisted vaginal hysterectomy, bilateral salpingectomy, and oophorectomy?

a. 58554
b. 58533, 58661-50
c. 58544
d. 58544, 58661-50

28. Code assignment for medical conditions is usually based on documentation by the patient's provider. Which of the following conditions may be documented by a clinician other than the patient's provider?

a. Elevated blood pressure
b. Obesity
c. Laterality
d. Nonpressure ulcer

29. What is the correct anesthesia code assignment for the revision of a total hip replacement?

a. 01200
b. 01214
c. 01210
d. 01215

30. What is the correct code assignment for an automated urinalysis with microscopy to detect protein?

a. 81000
b. 81003
c. 81001
d. 81002

31. What is the correct code assignment for a new 36-year-old female patient presenting for an annual gynecological examination?

a. 99385
b. 99395, 99459
c. 99395
d. 99385, 99459

32. What is the correct code assignment for a flexible transoral esophagogastroduodenoscopy with bougie dilation of the esophageal strictures?

a. 43249
b. 43245
c. 43233
d. 43266

33. What is the correct code assignment for intramuscular injection of heat-treated rabies immune globulin?

a. 90376, 96372
b. 96372, 90376
c. 90377
d. 90376

34. When can the CPT modifier -2P be assigned?

a. The procedure is contraindicated.
b. The patient declined the service.
c. Inadequate resources are available.
d. The patient already received the service.

35. Assign the correct diagnosis and procedure codes for the following encounter.

A 12-year-old female taking carbamazepine is brought by her mother for a follow-up for complex partial seizure disorder. The prior clinic notes were reviewed. A medically appropriate history and exam was performed. There have been no reported seizures since the carbamazepine was prescribed. There are no signs of toxicity found during her physical examination. The patient and her mother are counseled about her diagnosis of epilepsy and about seizure precautions, particularly during the school day. The mother is instructed to schedule a follow-up appointment for 3 months from now and to call the office in the interim if she has any questions or concerns. The provider spent 13 minutes counseling the patient and her mother for a total of 24 minutes for this encounter.

a. G40.409, 99123
b. G40.209, 99202
c. G40.409, 99202
d. G40.209, 99213

36. What is the correct code assignment for a 28-minute visit for an established patient residing in an assisted living facility?

a. 99341
b. 99347
c. 99308
d. 99304

37. What is the correct code assignment for a 3 mcg per 0.3 mL dose of an intramuscular vaccine against SARS-CoV-2 mRNA-lipid nanoparticle spiked protein?

a. 91320, 90480
b. 91322, 90480
c. 90480, 91318
d. 91318, 90480

38. What is the correct code assignment for total thyroidectomy for malignancy?

a. 60240
b. 60254
c. 60252
d. 60270

39. What is the correct code assignment for laparoscopic repair of a recurrent, incarcerated ventral hernia, including mesh implantation of a 6.0 cm defect?

a. 49616
b. 49594
c. 49622
d. 49615

40. What is borborygmus?

a. Discharge of fat in the feces
b. Black, tarry stools
c. Noise caused by gas moving through the intestine
d. Twisting of the intestine upon itself

41. What is the correct code assignment for a complete full-mouth radiological examination?

a. 70310
b. 70320
c. 70350
d. 70260

42. What is the function of the superior vena cava?

a. It drains blood from the upper part of the body.
b. It carries oxygen-rich blood to the right atrium.
c. It forms a passage to keep blood flowing in one direction.
d. It provides newly oxygenated blood to the left atrium.

43. What is the correct code assignment for a wraparound bone graft procedure including microvascular anastomosis of the right great toe?

a. 26551-T5
b. 20962-T5
c. 20973-T5
d. 20900-T5

44. What is the correct code assignment for nucleic acid detection of SARS-CoV-2 using the amplified probe technique?

a. 87637
b. 87635
c. 87636
d. 86413

45. What is the correct code assignment for an ERCP with lithotripsy destruction of calculus from the biliary duct?

a. 43275
b. 43264
c. 43265
d. 47544

46. A surgeon performs a wide local excision of a melanoma of the right mid-foot. The surgeon measures the lesion as 0.75 cm in diameter. He notes that the excision includes a margin of 1 cm on each side of the lesion. After the lesion is removed, the edges of the wound are reapproximated. The specimen is sent to pathology. The patient is given instructions for home care and is advised to return for suture removal in 7 days. What is the correct code assignment?

a. 11601
b. 11603
c. 11623
d. 11621

47. What is the correct code assignment for an anterovertical hemilaryngectomy?

a. 31380
b. 31382
c. 31370
d. 31375

48. What is the correct code assignment for total serum cholesterol, HDL cholesterol, and triglycerides?

a. 80061
b. 82465, 83718, 84478
c. 82465, 84478
d. 82705

49. A patient presents to the clinic for an intrauterine device (IUD) placement. A consent form is signed, and the provider successfully inserts a 19.5-mg levonorgestrel-releasing IUD. Assign the correct HCPCS Level II code.

a. S4989
b. J7296
c. S4981
d. J7298

50. What is the correct code assignment for laser fulguration and biopsy via cystourethroscopy of a 0.4-cm bladder tumor?

a. 52224
b. 52204
c. 52234
d. 52214

51. What does the combining form of *lept/o-* mean?

a. Thickened or hardened tissue
b. Smooth muscle
c. White or whiteness
d. Thin or slender

52. In skeletal anatomy, what is a *facet*?

a. A small, smooth, flat articular surface
b. A narrow, elongated elevation
c. A branchlike extension
d. A thornlike projection

53. Where is the spleen located?

a. Left lower quadrant of the abdomen
b. Left upper quadrant of the abdomen
c. Right upper quadrant of the abdomen
d. Perpendicular to the stomach

54. What phrase is included in the title of most manifestation codes in the ICD-10-CM tabular list?

a. In diseases classified elsewhere
b. Not elsewhere classified
c. Not otherwise specified
d. Unspecified disease

55. Assign the correct diagnosis and procedure codes for the following encounter.

A patient presents to the emergency department with acute chest pain. A 12-lead electrocardiogram shows ST-segment elevations, and blood work shows that the troponin level is elevated. An IV of D5NS is started to keep the vein open. Streptokinase is administered via IV by the physician for the ST elevation myocardial infarction. The patient is transferred to the critical care unit after 42 minutes of direct physician care in the emergency department. Medical decision-making was documented at a high level.

a. I21.3, 99285, 93000-PC, 92977
b. I21.9, 99291, 93000, 92977
c. I21.9, 99285, 92977
d. I21.3, 99291, 92977

56. What external-cause code category takes precedence over all other external-cause code categories?

a. Hurricane
b. Cataclysmic events
c. Flood
d. Elder abuse

57. What organization is the main enforcer of HIPAA rules?

a. Centers for Medicare and Medicaid Services
b. Office of Inspector General
c. Office for Civil Rights
d. Health Resources and Services Administration

58. What are the parathyroid glands?

a. Endocrine glands that release secretions to mobilize calcium into the bloodstream
b. Endocrine glands that secrete calcitonin when calcium levels are high
c. Small exocrine glands located at the vaginal orifice
d. Endocrine glands that secrete digestive enzymes into the gastrointestinal tract

59. A patient is seen in the emergency department and determined to be experiencing hallucinations due to drinking an unknown amount of alcohol. Assign the correct ICD-10-CM code for the encounter.

a. F10.151
b. F10.251
c. F10.121
d. F10.951

60. What is the correct code assignment for a cleft lip repair with a cross-lip pedicle flap, including sectioning and insertion of the pedicle?

a. 40761
b. 40700
c. 40701
d. 40527

61. A patient has a 3.5-cm^2 malignant lesion removed from his right cheek, which creates a 6.0-cm^2 defect. The area is immediately repaired with an advancement flap. What is the correct code assignment for this encounter?

a. 14060
b. 11646
c. 14040
d. 11644

62. What is the correct code assignment for a one-piece LeFort I procedure requiring bone grafts?

a. 21141
b. 21155
c. 21160
d. 21145

63. Assign the correct diagnosis and procedure codes for the following discharge note/management.

Discharge Note: A 54-year-old obese male patient, who has trouble ambulating, was admitted to the hospital via the emergency department due to a 1-week history of a dry cough, nausea, generalized aches and chills, temperature of 102.1 °F, shortness of breath, and labored breathing. A chest x-ray revealed patchy consolidation and ground-glass opacities consistent with ARDS. A subsequent nasopharyngeal swab tested positive for COVID-19. Today (Day 6), after passive oxygen therapy and antiviral treatment, the patient is released home. The patient lives alone and continues to require oxygen, so he will be receiving follow-up visits by home healthcare workers. His daughter is unable to stay at his house but will visit as often as possible. She will take him to his doctor visits and manage his medical care whenever possible. The daughter is to make an appointment for him with his primary care physician as well as one with the pulmonologist. The patient is to call the clinic if his symptoms increase or if he has trouble breathing. On the last day of the hospital stay, 24 minutes were spent counseling the patient and his daughter. An additional 10 minutes were spent reviewing the test results and progress notes.

a. U07.1, J80, E66.9, R26.2 99239
b. J80, U07.1, E66.01. R26.89, R50.9, 99239
c. U07.1, J80, E66.9, R26.89, 99238
d. U07.1, J98.8, E66.01, R26.2, R50.9, 99238

64. A patient presents to the dermatologist for biopsies of two lesions. The lesions are located on the left shoulder and the upper back on the left side. The left shoulder requires a punch biopsy. An incisional biopsy is performed on the back lesion. Assign the correct codes for this encounter.

a. 11104, 11105
b. 11105, 11104
c. 11105, 11106
d. 11106, 11105

65. A patient with worsening plantar fasciitis of the right foot is scheduled in the orthopedic clinic for a single injection. Assign the correct code(s) for the encounter.

a. 99212-25, 20550-RT
b. 20550-RT
c. 99213-25, 20550-RT
d. 20551-RT

66. What is the correct code assignment for secondary repair of the zone II flexor tendon, with a free graft?

a. 26350
b. 26358
c. 26357
d. 26356

67. What is the correct code assignment for a surgical nasal sinus endoscopy with an anterior and posterior ethmoidectomy including a sphenoidotomy?

a. 31255
b. 31243
c. 31259
d. 31257

68. What is the correct code assignment for a CT scan of the thoracic spine without contrast followed by a scan with contrast?

a. 72130
b. 72128, 72129
c. 72129, 72128
d. 72129

69. Assign the correct diagnosis and procedure codes for the following encounter.

A 75-year-old female patient, post–surgical hysterectomy 15 years prior, now has a third-degree vaginal vault prolapse. She is taken to the operating suite to have a colpocleisis performed.

Procedure Note: In the dorsal lithotomy position, the patient was prepped and draped under general anesthesia. The vault was grasped with two Allis clamps and completely externalized. A rectangular wedge of vaginal mucosa was transected both anteriorly and posteriorly until approximately 1 cm from the urethral meatus as well as 1 cm from the posterior fourchette. The vaginal mucosa was removed and discarded, after which the defect was reapproximated along the mucosal edges using several interrupted 1-0 Vicryl sutures. With the defect completely reduced, we proceeded to do a small perineorrhaphy. A wedge of perineovaginal skin was incised with Mayo scissors after instilling with 1% lidocaine with epinephrine. The vaginal mucosa was then reapproximated with 2-0 Vicryl in a running locked fashion, which was also used for the perineal muscles and overlying perineal skin. At this point, a Foley catheter was inserted, draining clear urine. Anesthesia was reversed, and the patient was transferred to recovery in stable condition. Estimated blood loss was approximated at 100 mL. There were no complications.

a. N18.9, Z90.710, 57282
b. N99.3, Z90.710, 57110
c. N99.3, Z90.710, 57120
d. N81.3, Z90.711, 5712

70. A 52-year-old female has undergone a mastectomy of her left breast with immediate placement of a tissue expander. The tissue expander ruptures unexpectedly. The surgeon examines the patient and recommends proceeding with a permanent left breast implant. The patient agrees, and the surgery is performed the following week. Assign the correct code for this procedure.

a. 11970-LT
b. 11960-LT
c. 19342-LT
d. 19330-LT

71. Assign the correct diagnosis and procedure codes for the following encounter.

A 12-year-old male patient presented to the emergency department with an injury to the left wrist after falling down the basement stairs. Radiographs confirmed a displaced fracture of the distal radius. The fracture was reduced under fluoroscopy with proper alignment shown in the postreduction x-ray. A cast was applied. The patient's mother was instructed to follow up with an orthopedic surgeon next week. She will contact their health insurance company for a list of in-network physicians. The patient was discharged from the emergency department in stable condition, and the mother was given fracture care instructions.

a. S52.592A, W10.9XXA, 25605-54-LT
b. S52.502A, W10.9XXA, 25605-54-LT
c. S52.502A, W10.9XXA, 25600-57-LT
d. S52.592A, W10.9XXA, 25600-57-LT

72. Assign the correct diagnosis and procedure codes for the following global pregnancy care.

A 39-year-old G2P1 patient at 39 weeks of gestation reports to labor and delivery for induction of labor after a previous Cesarean section. Membranes are ruptured and labor is induced via IV Pitocin. A healthy baby girl is delivered after 4.5 hours of labor. At 2 hours postdelivery, the patient's blood pressure drops, and a stat hemoglobin is 9.5 g/dL, down from an initial level of 11.0 g/dL. The physician returns to the recovery room and diagnoses a postpartum hemorrhage. The patient is transfused with 2 units of packed red blood cells, and "first line" conservative management protocol is followed, using oxytocin, methylergonovine maleate, and external uterine massage. Nursing staff is to contact the physician immediately with any adverse changes.

a. O09.513, Z3A.39, O34.211, O72.2, 59610
b. O09.523, O34.219, O72.1, 59614
c. O09.523, Z3A.39, O34.219, O72.1, 59610
d. O09.513, O34.211, O72.1, 59610

73. What is the correct code assignment for an anteroposterior colporrhaphy repair with mesh and a cystourethroscopy?

a. 57240, 57250-59, 57267
b. 57260, 52000
c. 57250, 57250-59, 52000
d. 57260, 57267

74. What is the correct anesthesia code assignment for an upper-abdomen incisional hernia repair?

a. 00756
b. 00750
c. 00752
d. 00832

75. Assign the correct diagnosis and procedure codes for the following encounter.

A 43-year-old male former football player, with left knee osteoarthritis due to a previous traumatic injury, reports to the orthopedic office for an injection of hylan G-F 20. The site is prepped with betadine, and 1% lidocaine is used for local anesthesia. An 18-gauge needle is inserted into the joint space, and synovial fluid is aspirated. The hylan G-F 20 is then injected intra-articularly. The patient is instructed to flex and extend the knee several times. Local compression is applied briefly, and a sterile bandage is placed on the injection site. The patient is to avoid any knee strain for at least 48 hours. An ice pack on the knee may be used for 10-minute intervals for pain and/or swelling. The patient should experience pain relief within 1–4 weeks. He is instructed to call the office if there are any adverse side effects.

a. M17.12, 20610-LT
b. M17.32, 20610-LT
c. M17.5, 20611-LT
d. M17.9, 20611-LT

76. What is the correct code assignment for ultrasonic placental location(s) for a twin pregnancy?

a. 76811, 76812
b. 76801, 76802
c. 76816
d. 76815

77. What is the correct code assignment for a consultation performed in a nursing facility and documented as 45 minutes in duration?

a. 99244
b. 99253
c. 99234
d. 99221

78. What does the combining form *sider/o-* mean?

a. Irregular
b. Iron
c. Pulse
d. Blue

79. What is the correct code assignment for open treatment of an orbital blowout fracture with a periorbital approach and bone graft?

a. 21386
b. 21390
c. 21395
d. 21385

80. According to CPT guidelines, which of the following is included with antepartum care?

a. Diagnostic laboratory testing
b. A 20-week ultrasound
c. Monthly visits to 28 weeks
d. Weekly visits after 28 weeks

81. What is the correct code assignment for *BRCA2* gene analysis of a known familial variant?

a. 81215
b. 81216
c. 81163
d. 81217

82. What is the correct code assignment for 18 minutes of counseling and risk factor reduction intervention, including healthy diet and exercise advice, provided to an established patient by a nurse practitioner?

a. 99078
b. 99408
c. 99407
d. 99401

83. What is the correct code assignment for a home visit by a nonphysician professional for assistance with activities of daily living and personal care?

a. 99509
b. 97535
c. 99600
d. 97530

84. What is the correct code assignment for the daily subsequent intensive care of a 2,500 g neonate?

a. 99479
b. 99480
c. 99469
d. 99478

85. What is the correct code assignment for continuous overnight monitoring of oxygen saturation via noninvasive pulse oximetry?

a. 94760
b. 94761
c. 94618
d. 94762

86. What is the correct code assignment for 30 minutes of psychotherapeutic counseling with a review of medication and refills of the patient's prescriptions of Wellbutrin and Vyvanse?

a. 90833, 90863
b. 90875
c. 90832, 90863
d. 90792

87. A patient presents to the office for laser ablation of a single 2-cm benign lesion of the right hand. Assign the correct code for this encounter.

a. 17110
b. 11402
c. 11422
d. 11307

88. What is the correct code assignment for epidural lumbar injection of alcohol for neurolysis?

a. 62280
b. 62292
c. 62282
d. 62320

89. What is the correct code assignment for colposcopy of the cervix with endocervical curettage, conization of the cervix, and endometrial biopsy?

a. 57456, 58110-59, 57461
b. 57456, 58110-59
c. 57461, 57456-59, 58110-59
d. 57461, 58110-59

90. What is the correct code assignment for bilateral repair of blepharoptosis using the frontalis muscle technique with banked fascia?

a. 67902-50
b. 67901-50
c. 67906-50
d. 67691-50

91. What is the correct code assignment for an intravenous pyelogram of the kidney, ureter, and bladder with tomography of the renal pelvis?

a. 74018
b. 74019
c. 74400
d. 74150

92. What is the correct code assignment for a video-assisted thoracoscopic surgery with excision of a mediastinal tumor?

a. 32661
b. 32666
c. 32662
d. 32503

93. What does the OIG-issued General Compliance Program Guidance recommend that small entities include in their annual audit?

a. Assessment of any overpayments
b. Reporting of provider bonuses
c. Applicable workers' compensation exclusion lists
d. Additional audits by an outside contractor

94. A 30-year-old male is seen in the emergency department after suffering a traumatic 6.75-cm jagged laceration to his left forearm due to a chainsaw accident. The area is cleaned, and the physician debrides nonviable tissue at the edges of the wound prior to a layered closure. What is the correct code assignment for this encounter?

a. 12034
b. 13121
c. 12042
d. 13132

95. What is the correct anesthesia code assignment for a cataract removal?

a. 00142
b. 00140
c. 00144
d. 00145

96. What is the correct code assignment for intracranial neuroendoscopy for transnasal excision of a pituitary tumor?

a. 62161
b. 62165
c. 62162
d. 62164

97. A patient presents for a preprocedural ultrasound of benign uterine fibroids prior to a supracervical hysterectomy. What is the correct ICD-10 code assignment for this encounter?

a. D25.9, Z01.818
b. Z01.818, D25.1
c. Z01.89, D25.1
d. Z01.818, D25.9

98. What is the correct code assignment for a cervical cytopathology automated thin layer prep Pap smear with manual screening under physician supervision?

a. 88174
b. 88143
c. 88142
d. 88175

99. What is the correct code assignment for bilateral laminectomy of L1 and L2 with decompression of the nerve roots?

a. 63047-RT, 63047-LT, 63048-50
b. 63042, 63044-50
c. 63042, 63044-RT, 63044-LT
d. 63047, 63048

100. What is the correct code assignment for a radiological exam including a single view of the chest and a complete acute abdomen series in both the erect position and the supine position?

a. 74022
b. 71045, 74021
c. 74021, 71045
d. 74019

Answer Key and Explanations for Test #1

1. D: Code 47382 is assigned from the Liver, Other Procedures category in the Digestive System section. Using the CPT index, this can be found with the following:

Liver
  Ablation
    Tumor: 47380–47383

The tabular section descriptions are then reviewed to assign the correct code.

2. A: The compliance committee charter should include a statement of purpose, scope, roles and responsibilities, membership, meeting frequency, and other functions of the compliance committee. The guidance does not reference salaries or clinical nursing assessments. The guidance also states that a formal disclosure program may not be necessary or appropriate for a small organization.

3. D: CPT evaluation and management guidelines for codes 99242–99255 state that consultations initiated by a patient or family are not reported using the consultation codes. Only those consultations requested by a physician, other qualified healthcare professional, or other appropriate source (e.g., a social worker, educator, lawyer, or insurance company) are reported using the consultation codes.

4. B: Code 80307 is assigned from the Non-Specific Drug Screening category in the Pathology and Laboratory section. Using the CPT index, this can be found with the following:

Screening, Drug (see Drug Screen)
  Drug Screen
    Mass Spectrometry: 80307
    Chromatography: 80307

5. B: Code 93580 is assigned from the Percutaneous Repair of Congenital Heart Defects category in the Medicine section. Using the CPT index, this can be found with the following:

Congenital Cardiac Anomaly/Defect
  Atrial Septal Defect
    Closure: 33675–33677, 93580

The tabular section descriptions are then reviewed to assign the correct code.

6. C: Code 52601 is assigned from the Vesical Neck and Prostate category in the Urinary System section. The coding instructions beneath 52601 state that for a first-stage transurethral partial resection of the prostate, use code 52601.

7. D: The ileum is the third part of the small intestine, and it connects to the cecum. It helps to further digest food from the stomach and other parts of the small intestine. The ilium is the uppermost and largest part of the pelvic girdle. The sacrum is a triangular bone that is the posterior skeletal element forming the pelvis.

8. A: First, search the ICD-10 index for the following:

Carcinoma
  Basal Cell: C44.91 (see also Skin, Malignant)

From the neoplasm table:

Malignant
  Primary
    Skin
      Scalp
        Basal Cell
          Carcinoma: C44.41

Second, confirm the ICD-10-CM code by reviewing the description in the tabular list to ensure that the appropriate code is selected. The narrative description for C44.41 is "Basal cell carcinoma of the skin of the scalp and neck."

Code 11624 is assigned from the Excision, Malignant Lesions category in the Surgery/Integumentary section. Using the CPT index, this can be found with the following:

Excision
  Lesion
    Skin
      Malignant: 11620–11624, 11626, 11640–11644, 11646

The tabular section descriptions are then reviewed to assign the correct code for the location and size. There is a Code Also note at codes 11600–11646 for Reconstruction (graft) procedure.

Code 15100 is assigned from the Autografts category in the Surgery/Integumentary section. Using the CPT index, this can be found with the following:

Graft
  Skin
    Split Graft: 15100, 15101, 15120, 15121

The tabular section descriptions are then reviewed to assign the correct code. The modifier -51 is appended to indicate that multiple procedures were performed.

9. D: Code 33776 is assigned from the Repair Aberrant Anatomy: Transposition of Great Vessels category in the Cardiovascular, Hemic, and Lymphatic section. Using the CPT index, this can be found with the following:

Transposition
  Great Arteries
    Repair: 33770–33781

The tabular section descriptions are then reviewed to assign the correct code.

10. D: First, search the HCPCS index for *surgical stocking* and find codes A4490–A4510. Note that there are additional entries for *stocking, gradient compression*, which are coded in categories A6530–A6549, A6552–A6564, and A6610. Then, search the tabular list to select full-length surgical stockings. The correct code assignment is A4510 (surgical stockings, full-length, each).

11. B: The ICD-10-CM Guidelines (see I.C. g. [1] [j]) indicate that patients who are being seen for follow-up examination of COVID-19 and are asymptomatic and no longer test positive will be assigned code Z09 (encounter for follow-up examination after completed treatment for conditions other than malignant neoplasm). Then, they are assigned Z86.16, personal history of COVID-19 (note the sequencing of diagnosis codes). Code U09.9 is incorrect because it describes post-COVID-19 condition, unspecified.

12. C: First, search the ICD-10 index for the following:

Arthritis
  Traumatic
    Left Hip: M12.552

Then, confirm the code in the tabular list.

13. A: First, search the ICD-10 index for the following:

Diabetes, Type 2: E11.9
Hypertension: I10
Overweight: E66.3
Body Mass Index
  Adult
    35.0–35.9: Z68.35

Second, confirm all of the ICD-10-CM codes by reviewing the descriptions in the tabular list to ensure that the appropriate codes are selected.

Code 99214 is assigned from the Outpatient and Other Visits in the Evaluation and Management section. Using the CPT index, this can be found with the following:

Evaluation and Management Services
  Office/Outpatient: 99201–99215

The tabular section descriptions are then reviewed to assign the correct code.

14. B: Code 78351 is assigned from the Nuclear Radiology, Bones and Joints category in the Radiology section. Using the CPT index, this can be found with the following:

Absorptiometry
  Dual Photon
    Bone: 78351

15. A: First, search the ICD-10 index for the following:

Syndrome
  HELLP: O14.2-

Then, search the tabular list to correctly assign O14.25 (HELLP syndrome complicating the puerperium). The ICD-10-CM includes notes state "severe preeclampsia with hemolysis, elevated liver enzymes, and low platelet count." ICD-10-CM codes O14.95, O14.15, and O14.05 describe the condition of preeclampsia only.

16. B: Codes 29827-RT and 29824-51-RT are assigned from the Endoscopy/Arthroscopy category in the Musculoskeletal System section. Using the CPT index, this can be found with the following:

Arthroscopy
  Surgical
    Shoulder: 29806–29828

The tabular section descriptions are then reviewed to assign the correct code. CPT code 29827 describes an arthroscopic rotator cuff repair. The instructional notes state "when an arthroscopic distal clavicle resection is performed at the same setting, use code 29824 and append modifier -51 to indicate that multiple procedures were performed." Modifier -RT, as described in CPT Appendix A, is included with codes 29827 and 29824 to indicate that each procedure was performed on the right side. In this case, it is appended as a second modifier to CPT code 29824 because modifier -51 will impact reimbursement and modifier -RT is an informational site designation modifier that does not impact reimbursement.

17. B: First, search the ICD-10 index for the following:

Calculus
  Urinary Tract
    With Hydronephrosis: N13.2

Second, confirm the ICD-10-CM code by reviewing the description in the tabular list to ensure that the appropriate code is selected. The narrative description for N13.2 is "Hydronephrosis with renal and ureteral obstruction," but ICD-10-CM guidance states that *and* means *and/or*. The fever is not assigned because an elevated temperature is an integral symptom of hydronephrosis.

Code 74150 is assigned from the Computed Tomography, Abdomen category in the Radiology section. Code 99284 is assigned from the Emergency Department Visits category in the Evaluation and Management section. Using the CPT index, this can be found with the following:

Evaluation and Management Services
  Emergency Department: 99281–99285

18. B: Code 50382 is assigned from the Renal Pelvis Catheter Procedures category in the Urinary System chapter. This encounter is for the removal and replacement of an indwelling ureteral stent via a percutaneous approach. The radiology portion is included in the code description. Codes 50384 and 50386 are for removal only. Code 50385 is performed via a transurethral approach.

Using the CPT index, this can be found with the following:

Stent
  Replacement
    Ureteral: 50382

19. B: Code 30450 is assigned from the Reconstruction or Repair of the Nose category in the Respiratory System section. Using the CPT index, this can be found with the following:

Rhinoplasty
  Secondary: 30430–30450

The tabular section descriptions are then reviewed to assign the correct code.

20. B: Coding guidelines for obstetrics cases require codes from Chapter 15, codes in the range O00–O9A, Pregnancy, Childbirth, and the Puerperium. Chapter 15 codes have sequencing priority over codes from other chapters. Additional codes from other chapters may be used in conjunction with Chapter 15 codes to further specify conditions. This includes COVID-19 cases during pregnancy, childbirth, or the puerperium; when COVID-19 is the reason for the admission or encounter, code O98.5-. Other viral diseases complicating pregnancy, childbirth, and the puerperium should be sequenced as the principal/first-listed diagnosis; code U07.1, COVID-19, and the appropriate codes for associated manifestation(s) should be assigned as additional diagnoses. During pregnancy, childbirth, or the puerperium, a patient admitted (or presenting for a healthcare encounter) because of an HIV-related illness should receive a principal diagnosis code of O98.7-, Human immunodeficiency virus disease complicating pregnancy, childbirth, and the puerperium, followed by B20 and the code(s) for the HIV-related illness(es). Patients with asymptomatic HIV infection status admitted (or presenting for a healthcare encounter) during pregnancy, childbirth, or the puerperium should receive codes of O98.7- and Z21.

21. B: Code 31631 is assigned from the Endoscopy of Lung category in the Respiratory System section. Using the CPT index, this can be found with the following:

Bronchoscopy
  Stent Placement: 31631, 31636, 31637

The tabular section descriptions are then reviewed to assign the correct code.

22. A: Code 66988-LT is assigned from the Intraocular Lens Procedure category in the Eye and Ocular Adnexa chapter. Using the CPT index, this can be found with the following:

Cataract
  Extraction/Removal
    Extracapsular
      With Endoscopic Cyclophotocoagulation: 66987, 66988

The tabular section descriptions are then reviewed to assign the correct code. Refer to CPT Appendix A for descriptions of the modifiers.

23. A: First, search the HCPCS index for splint, digit, prefabricated, to find code S8450. The instructional note states to specify which digit by using a modifier. The -F6 modifier is right hand, second digit. Code Q4049 is for finger splint, static. The HCPCS code A4570 is for an unspecified splint.

24. D: Code 45390 is assigned from the Colon and Rectum, Endoscopy category in the Digestive System section. Although a submucosal injection is performed, there is a note stating that 45381 is not to be reported with 45390 when it involves the same lesion. Using the CPT index, this can be found with the following:

Colonoscopy
  Flexible
    Mucosal Resection: 45390

25. B: Code 00404 is assigned from the Anesthesia for Chest/Pectoral Girdle Procedures category in the Anesthesia section. Using the CPT index, this can be found with the following:

Anesthesia
  Breast: 00402–00406

The tabular section descriptions are then reviewed to assign the correct code.

26. C: Code 99456 is assigned from the Life/Disability Insurance Eligibility Visits category in the Evaluation and Management section. Using the CPT index, this can be found with the following:

Evaluation and Management Services
  Disability/Work-Related Examination: 99450–99456

The tabular section descriptions are then reviewed to assign the correct code.

27. A: Code 58554 is assigned from the Corpus Uteri, Laparoscopy/Hysteroscopy category in the Female Genital System chapter. Using the CPT index, this can be found in a few different ways:

Laparoscopy
  Hysterectomy: 58541–58544, 58570–58575

or

Hysterectomy
  Vaginal: 58260–58270, 58290–58294, 58550–58544

or

Hysterectomy
  Vaginal
    Removal of Tubes
      Ovaries: 58562, 58263, 58291, 58292, 58552, 58554

The tabular section descriptions are then reviewed to assign the correct code.

28. C: General Coding Guideline I.B.14 indicates that code assignment is based on the documentation by the patient's provider (i.e., the physician or other qualified health-care practitioner legally accountable for establishing the patient's diagnosis). There are a few exceptions when code assignment may be based on medical record documentation from clinicians who are not the patient's provider. In this context, the phrase "clinicians other than the patient's provider" refers to healthcare professionals permitted, based on regulatory or accreditation requirements or internal hospital policies, to document in a patient's official medical record. These exceptions include codes for the following:

- Body mass index
- Depth of non-pressure chronic ulcers
- Pressure ulcer stage
- Coma scale
- National Institutes of Health Stroke Scale
- Social determinants of health
- Laterality

- Blood alcohol level
- Underimmunization status

29. D: Code 01215 is assigned from the Anesthesia for Lower Extremity Procedures category in the Anesthesia section. Using the CPT index, this can be found with the following:

Anesthesia
  Arthroplasty
    Hip: 01214, 01215

The tabular section descriptions are then reviewed to assign the correct code.

30. C: Code 81001 is assigned from the Urine Tests category in the Pathology and Laboratory section. Using the CPT index, this can be found with the following:

Urinalysis
  Automated: 81001, 81003

The tabular section descriptions are then reviewed to assign the correct code.

31. D: Code 99385 is assigned from the Preventive Medicine Visits category in the Evaluation and Management section. Using the CPT index, this can be found with the following:

Evaluation and Management Services
  Preventive Medicine Services: 99381–99429

The tabular section descriptions are then reviewed to assign the correct code. There is an instructional note that states to also code a pelvic examination, when performed (99459). At 99459, there is a code-first note: 99383–99387.

32. B: Code 43245 is assigned from the Endoscopic Procedures, Esophagogastroduodenoscopy category in the Digestive System section. Using the CPT index, this can be found with the following:

Esophagogastroduodenoscopy (EGD)
  Flexible Transoral
    Dilation of Esophagus: 43233, 43249

The tabular section descriptions are then reviewed to assign the correct code.

33. A: Code 90376 is assigned from the Immunoglobulin Products category in the Medicine section. Using the CPT index, this can be found with the following:

Immune Globulins
  Rabies
    Rabies Immune Globulin, Heat-treated (RIgH): 90376

There is an instructional note at 90281–90399 to also code 96365–96372, 96374–96375. The tabular section descriptions are then reviewed to assign the correct code. Assign code 96372 for therapeutic, prophylactic, or diagnostic injection, intramuscular or subcutaneous.

34. B: Modifier -2P is a Category II code. It can be assigned when the patient declines services for economic, social, religious, or other patient reasons. Modifier -1P is assigned when a procedure is contraindicated or when the service has already been received. Modifier -3P indicates that the resources to perform the service are unavailable.

35. D: First, search the ICD-10 index for the following:

Seizure(s)
  Partial
    Complex (see Epilepsy, Localization-related, Symptomatic, With Complex Partial Seizures)
Epilepsy
  Localization-related (focal) (partial)
    Symptomatic
      With Complex Partial Seizures: G40.209

Second, confirm the ICD-10-CM code by reviewing the description in the tabular list to ensure that the appropriate code is selected.

Code 99213 is assigned from the Outpatient and Other Visits category in the Evaluation and Management section. Using the CPT index, this can be found with the following:

Evaluation and Management Services
  Office/Outpatient: 99202–99215

The tabular section descriptions are then reviewed to assign the correct code.

36. B: Code 99347 is assigned from the Home and Residence Visits category in the Evaluation and Management section. Using the CPT index, this can be found with the following:

Evaluation and Management Services
  Home or Residence: 99341–99350

The tabular section descriptions are then reviewed to assign the correct code.

37. D: Code 91318 is assigned from the Vaccine/Toxoid Products category in the Medicine section. Using the CPT index, this can be found with the following:

Vaccines
  Severe Acute Respiratory Syndrome: 91304, 91318, 91319, 91320, 91321, 91322

The tabular section descriptions are then reviewed to assign the correct code. There is an instructional note at 91318 to also code vaccine administration. Assign code 90480 for immunization administration by intramuscular injection of COVID-19 vaccine, single dose.

38. A: Code 60240 is assigned from the Thyroid Gland category in the Endocrine System chapter. Using the CPT index, this can be found with the following:

Thyroidectomy, Total: 60240, 60271

The tabular section descriptions are then reviewed to assign the correct code. Code 60240 applies to any total thyroidectomy, regardless of malignancy.

39. A: Code 49616 is assigned from the Repair, Hernioplasty, Herniorrhaphy, Herniotomy category in the Digestive System section. Using the CPT index, this can be found with the following:

Hernia
  Repair
    Ventral: 49591–49596, 49613, 49614, 49615, 49616, 49617, 49618

The tabular section descriptions are then reviewed to assign the correct code.

40. C: Borborygmus is the rumbling, gurgling noise caused by gas moving through the intestine and is considered a normal part of the digestion process. Steatorrhea is the passage of fat into the feces due to the failure to digest and absorb it. It can occur in pancreatic disease and malabsorption syndromes. Melena is black, tarry stool caused by internal bleeding, typically of the upper gastrointestinal tract. Volvulus is twisting of the intestines, which causes an obstruction; left untreated, it may result in vascular compromise of the site.

41. B: Code 70320 is assigned from the Head, Neck, and Orofacial Structures category in the Radiology section. Using the CPT index, this can be found with the following:

X-ray
  Teeth: 70300–70320

The tabular section descriptions are then reviewed to assign the correct code.

42. A: The superior vena cava is a large, valveless vein that conveys oxygen-poor venous blood from the upper half of the body and returns it to the right atrium. The pulmonary veins are the only veins that carry oxygen-rich blood from the lungs to the heart. They provide blood to the left atrium. The valves of the heart open and close tightly, maintaining blood flow in only one direction.

43. A: Code 26551-T5 is assigned from the Repair, Revision, and/or Reconstruction of Hands or Fingers category in the Musculoskeletal System section. Using the CPT index, this can be found with the following:

Graft
  Bone
    Microvascular: 20955–20962

CPT code 20973 has an instructional note stating, "for great toe wraparound procedure, use 26551." Modifier -T5, as described in CPT Appendix A, is included to indicate that the procedure was performed on the right great toe.

44. C: Code 87636 is assigned from the Infectious Agent Detection by Probe Technique category in the Pathology and Laboratory section. Using the CPT index, this can be found with the following:

COVID-19
  Infectious Agent Detection
    Nucleic Acid Probe Technique: 87635, 87636, 87637

The tabular section descriptions are then reviewed to assign the correct code.

45. C: Code 43265 is assigned from the Endoscopic Retrograde Cholangiopancreatography category in the Digestive System section. Using the CPT index, this can be found with the following:

Endoscopy
  Bile Duct
    Destruction
      Calculi (stone): 43265

46. C: Code 11623 for the removal of a melanoma would be coded as excision of a malignant lesion. The CPT instructions in the Excision, Malignant Lesions category of the Integumentary section state that the code is selected by measuring the greatest clinical diameter of the lesion plus the margin required for complete excision.

47. A: Code 31380 is assigned from the Procedures of the Larynx category in the Respiratory System section. Using the CPT index, this can be found with the following:

Laryngectomy
  Partial: 31367–31382

The tabular section descriptions are then reviewed to assign the correct code.

48. A: Code 80061 is assigned from the Multi-test Laboratory Panels category in the Pathology and Laboratory section. Using the CPT index, this can be found with the following:

Panel
  Organ or Disease-oriented Panel
    Lipid: 80061

49. B: First, search the HCPCS index for Levonorgestrel-Releasing Intrauterine Device to find the following codes: J7296–J7298, S4981. Then, search the tabular list. This requires selecting the correct dosage for a levonorgestrel-releasing IUD. Code J7296 is for the levonorgestrel-releasing IUD (Kyleena), 19.5 mg. Appendix 1, Table of Drugs, also includes Kyleena 19.5 mg. To accurately assign the code, the selection must be as specific as possible. The question states that the IUD dosage is 19.5 mg; therefore, J7296 is the correct answer.

Codes S4981 and S4989 are incorrect because the narrative description in the tabular section does not state an IUD with 19.5-mg dosage. These codes have a generic description. A levonorgestrel-releasing IUD with no dosage documented is S4981. Code S4989 does not state that the product is a levonorgestrel-releasing IUD.

50. A: Code 52224 is assigned from the Transurethral Surgery, Urethra and Bladder category in the Urinary System chapter. This encounter is for cystourethroscopy with fulguration of lesions less than 0.5 cm. The procedure description states that a biopsy may be included.

51. D: The combining form *lept/o-* means "thin" or "slender." A leptosome is a person with a small body frame and a slender physique. *Leiomyo-* means "smooth muscle tissue" and can cause uterine leiomyoma, also known as noncancerous fibroid tumors. The combining form *leuk/o-* means "white." Thickened or hardened tissue is described with the combining form *scler/o-*.

52. A: A facet is a small, smooth, flat articular surface of a bone. Examples of facets can be seen in the joints of the vertebrae, which allow for flexion and extension of the spine. A crest is a bony ridge such as the iliac crest of the ilium. A ramus is a branchlike extension that provides structural support to the rest of the bone; examples can be found on the mandible and pubic bones. A spine is a sharp or thornlike process of a bone; examples can be found on the cervical, thoracic, and lumbar vertebrae.

53. B: The spleen is a large, vascular lymphatic organ located in the left upper quadrant of the abdomen, adjacent to the stomach. It is not essential for life, but it does store blood, including platelets, and filter blood to remove abnormal cells.

54. A: ICD-10 Guidance I.A.13 states that tabular list manifestation codes will have the phrase "in diseases classified elsewhere" in the code title. Codes with this title are a component of the etiology/manifestation convention. "In diseases classified elsewhere" codes are never permitted to be used as first-listed or principal diagnosis codes. They must be used in conjunction with an underlying condition code, and they must be listed following the underlying condition.

The abbreviation NEC (not elsewhere classifiable) in the tabular list represents "other specified." When a diagnosis is specified but there is no code available for that diagnosis, the tabular list includes an NEC entry under a code to identify it as the "other specified" code. The abbreviation NOS (not otherwise specified) is the equivalent of the code for a condition that is unspecified. An example of this convention would be ICD-10-CM code R52: "Pain, unspecified."

55. D: First, search the ICD-10 index for the following:

Infarction
  ST Elevation (STEMI): I21.3

Second, confirm the ICD-10-CM code by reviewing the description in the tabular list to ensure that the appropriate code is selected.

Code 99291 is assigned from the Critical Care Visits 72 Months of Age or Older category in the Evaluation and Management section. Using the CPT index, this can be found with the following:

Evaluation and Management Services
  Critical Care: 99291, 99292

The critical care code is assigned based on time. Critical care is defined in the instructional notes as medical care of a critical condition or injury that acutely impairs one or more vital organ systems such that there is a high probability of imminent or life-threatening deterioration. Electrocardiograms are noted as included in critical care as part of the collection of physiological data, so they are not coded separately.

Administration of streptokinase for thrombolysis is not included in the list of services for critical care. Code 92977 is assigned from the Intravascular Coronary Procedures category in the Medicine Section. Using the CPT index, this can be found with the following:

Thrombolysis
  Coronary Vessels: 93975, 92977

The tabular section descriptions are then reviewed to assign the correct code.

56. D: Per ICD-10-CM Guideline I.B.19.b, codes for cataclysmic events, such as a flood or hurricane, take priority over most other external-cause codes and should be sequenced before the other codes. The exception is when the external cause is child or elder abuse or terrorism, in which case the abuse or terrorism takes priority.

57. C: HIPAA rules are predominantly enforced by the Office for Civil Rights, a division of the US Department of Health and Human Services (HHS). HHS is responsible for enhancing the health and well-being of all Americans by providing health and human services and by fostering sound, sustained advances in the sciences underlying medicine, public health, and social services. The Office of Inspector General is the division of HHS charged with fighting waste, fraud, and abuse and with improving the efficiency of Medicare, Medicaid, and more than 100 other HHS programs. The Centers for Medicare and Medicaid Services is a federal agency within HHS that provides healthcare coverage to more than 160 million people through Medicare, Medicaid, the Children's Health Insurance Program, and the Health Insurance Marketplace. The Health Resources and Services Administration, a division of HHS, provides healthcare to people who are geographically isolated or economically or medically vulnerable.

58. A: The parathyroid glands are endocrine glands that help mobilize calcium into the bloodstream. The thyroid gland secretes T3 and T4 hormones, both of which are necessary to maintain a normal level of metabolism in all body cells. The Bartholin's glands produce a mucous secretion that lubricates the vagina. The islets of Langerhans are specialized cells within the pancreas that produce the hormones insulin and glucagon.

59. D: First, search the ICD-10 index for the following:

Hallucinosis
  Alcoholic (acute): F10.951

There is an alternate index entry:

Alcohol, Alcoholic, Alcohol-induced
  Hallucinosis (acute): F10.951

In the tabular list, search for F10.951 and confirm the selection: alcohol use, unspecified with alcohol-induced psychotic disorder with hallucinations. Code F10.151 is for hallucinations/hallucinosis, alcoholic (acute) indicating abuse; code F10.251 is for hallucinations/hallucinosis, alcoholic (acute) indicating dependence; and code F10.121 is for alcohol abuse with intoxication delirium.

60. A: Code 40761 is assigned from the Resection and Repair Procedures of the Lip category in the Digestive System section. Using the CPT index, this can be found with the following:

Repair
  Lip
    Cleft Series: 40700–40761

The tabular section descriptions are then reviewed to assign the correct code.

61. C: CPT instructions in the Adjacent Tissue Transfer or Rearrangement of the Integumentary section state that codes 14000–14302 are used for excision (including lesion) and/or repair by adjacent tissue transfer or rearrangement (this includes an advancement flap). Repair of a defect in the cheek that is less than 10 cm^2 falls under code 14040. The excision of a malignant lesion (11600–11646) is not separately reportable with codes 14000–14302.

62. D: Code 21145 is assigned from the Repair, Revision and/or Reconstruction Head category in the Musculoskeletal System section. Using the CPT index, this can be found with the following:

LeFort I procedure
  Midface Reconstruction: 21141–21147

The tabular section descriptions are then reviewed to assign the correct code.

63. A: First, search the ICD-10 index for the following:

COVID-19: U07.1
Syndrome, Acute Respiratory Distress: J80
Obesity: E66.9
Difficult, Difficulty (in)
  Walking: R26.2

Second, confirm the ICD-10-CM codes by reviewing the description in the tabular list to ensure that the appropriate codes are selected. The guidelines for COVID-19 coding state that COVID-19 is sequenced first, followed by the appropriate codes for the associated manifestations.

Code 99239 is assigned from the Hospital Inpatient and Observation Services category in the Evaluation and Management section. Using the CPT index, this can be found with the following:

Evaluation and Management Services
  Discharge Management
    Inpatient or Observation Services: 99238–99239

The tabular section descriptions are then reviewed to assign the correct code. Per CPT instructions, discharge services are to be selected based on the total time spent.

64. D: Codes 11106 and 11105 are correct because CPT instructions in the Biopsy category of the Integumentary section state that when multiple biopsy techniques are performed during the same encounter, only one primary lesion code is reported. If an incisional biopsy is performed, report code 11106 in combination with a punch biopsy (code 11105).

65. B: Code 20550-RT is assigned from the Introduction or Removal category in the Musculoskeletal System section. CPT code 20550 uses "plantar fascia" in the code descriptor as an example of a condition being treated with the injection. Modifier -RT, as described in CPT Appendix A, is included to indicate that the procedure was performed on the right side. An evaluation and management service is not assigned because the injection is a planned procedure.

66. B: Code 26358 is assigned from the Repair, Revision and/or Reconstruction Hands or Fingers category in the Musculoskeletal System section. Using the CPT index, this can be found with the following:

Repair
  Tendon
    Flexor: 26350, 26352, and 26356–26358

The tabular section descriptions are then reviewed to assign the correct code.

67. D: Code 31257 is assigned from the Nasal Endoscopy with Ethmoid Removal category in the Respiratory System section. Using the CPT index, this can be found with the following:

Endoscopy
  Nose
    Surgical: 31237–31241, 31253–31257, 31259, 31267, 31276, 31287, 31288, 31290–31298

The tabular section descriptions are then reviewed to assign the correct code.

68. A: Code 72130 is assigned from the Computed Tomography, Thorax category in the Radiology section. Using the CPT index, this can be found with the following:

Bone
  With and Without Contrast
    Spine
      Thoracic: 72130

69. C: First, search the ICD-10 index for the following:

Prolapse
  Vagina
    Post-hysterectomy N99.3
Absence
  Uterus (acquired): Z90.710

Second, confirm the ICD-10-CM codes by reviewing the descriptions in the tabular list to ensure that the appropriate codes are selected.

Code 57120 is assigned from the Excisional Procedures: Vagina category in the Genital System section. Using the CPT index, this can be found with the following:

Colpocleisis: 57120

70. A: CPT instructions in the Mastectomy Procedures: Repair and Reconstruction category of the Integumentary section state that code 11970 describes the removal of a tissue expander with concurrent insertion of a permanent breast implant. Modifier -LT, as described in CPT Appendix A, is included to indicate that the procedure was performed on the left side.

71. B: First, search the ICD-10 index for the following:

Fracture
  Radius
    Distal End (see Fracture, Radius, Lower End)
      Lower End: S52.50-

Second, confirm the ICD-10-CM code by reviewing the description in the tabular list to ensure the laterality of the fracture (left) and the seventh character (A) that represents initial care. The appropriate code is S52.502A, unspecified fracture of the lower end of the left radius. There is an inclusion note at S52.5 that states "fracture of distal end of radius."

To assign the code for the fall, search the ICD-10 external-cause index for the following:

Fall
    Stairs, Steps: W10.9-

Then, confirm the ICD-10-CM external-cause code by reviewing the description in the tabular list. The description states that code W10.9 requires seven digits. Placeholder "X" is assigned twice, and "A" is assigned as an initial encounter. The appropriate code is W10.9XXA.

Code 25605-LT is assigned from the Treatment of Fracture/Dislocation of Forearm or Wrist category in the Musculoskeletal System section. Using the CPT index, this can be found with the following:

Fracture
    Radius
        Distal
            Closed: 25600–25605

The tabular section descriptions are then reviewed to assign the correct code for the manipulation/reduction of the fracture. Modifier -54 is assigned for the emergency department provider because only reduction of the fracture was provided and the patient will be seen by an orthopedic surgeon for follow-up. Modifier -LT identifies the left radius.

72. C: First, search the ICD-10 index for the following:

Pregnancy
    Supervision of
        Elderly Mother
            Multigravida: O09.52- (requires a sixth digit)
    Weeks of gestation
        39 Weeks: Z3A.39
    Cesarean Delivery, Previous, Affecting Management of Pregnancy: O34.219
    Hemorrhage
        Postpartum NEC (following delivery of placenta): O72.1

Second, confirm all of the ICD-10-CM codes by reviewing the description in the tabular list to ensure that the appropriate codes are selected.

Code 59610 is assigned from the Delivery after Previous Cesarean Delivery category in the Maternity Care and Delivery section. Using the CPT index, this can be found with the following:

Pregnancy
    Vaginal Delivery
        After Cesarean Section: 59610–59614

The tabular section descriptions are then reviewed to assign the correct code.

73. D: Code 57260 and add-on code 57267 are assigned from the Vagina, Repair category in the Female Genital System chapter. The procedure is a combined anteroposterior colporrhaphy. The cystourethroscopy is included per the code description. However, the mesh to reinforce the repair is an add-on code and is listed separately. The instructional note below code 57267 advises to use it in conjunction with codes 57240–57265.

74. C: Code 00752 is assigned from the Anesthesia for Abdominal Procedures category in the Anesthesia section. Using the CPT index, this can be found with the following:

Anesthesia
  Hernia Repair
    Abdomen
      Upper: 00750, 00752, 00756

The tabular section descriptions are then reviewed to assign the correct code.

75. B: First, search the ICD-10 index for the following:

Osteoarthritis
  Post-traumatic
    Knee: M17.3-

Second, confirm the ICD-10-CM code by reviewing the description in the tabular list to ensure that the appropriate code is selected. In this case, the laterality is left and therefore M17.32 is assigned.

Code 20610 is assigned from the Introduction or Removal category in the Surgery, Musculoskeletal section. Using the CPT index, this can be found with the following:

Injection
  Joint: 20600, 20604–20606, 20610, 20611

The tabular section descriptions are then reviewed to assign the correct code; refer to Appendix A for descriptions of the CPT modifiers.

76. D: Code 76815 is assigned from the Ultrasound, Other Fetal Evaluations category in the Radiology section. Using the CPT index, this can be found with the following:

Ultrasound
  Obstetrical
    Pregnant Uterus: 76801, 76802, 76805, 76810–76817

The tabular section descriptions are then reviewed to assign the correct code. Code 76815 states: Ultrasound, pregnant uterus, limited (placental location) 1 or more fetuses.

77. B: Code 99253 is assigned from the Consultations: Inpatient or Observation category in the Evaluation and Management section. Using the CPT index, this can be found with the following:

Evaluation and Management Services
  Consultations
    Inpatient or Observation: 99252–99255

The tabular section descriptions are then reviewed to assign the correct code. There is an instructional note that states that all consultations provided in hospital inpatient, observation, nursing facility, or partial hospitalization settings are included.

78. B: The combining form *sider/o-* means "iron." *Sideroblastic anemia* is a type of anemia that results from abnormal use of iron during erythropoiesis. The combining form for "irregular" or "varied" is *poikil/o-*. *Poikilocytosis* refers to an increase in abnormal red blood cells of any shape that comprise 10% or more of the total number of red blood cells. The combining form for "pulse" is *sphygm/o-* and is used in the term *sphygmomanometer*, an instrument used to measure the blood pressure. The combining form *cyan/o-* means "blue." *Cyanosis* refers to a bluish color appearing in the skin, lips, and nail beds, indicating a shortage of oxygen in the blood.

79. C: Code 21395 is assigned from the Fracture and/or Dislocation Head category in the Musculoskeletal System section. Using the CPT index, this can be found with the following:

Fracture
  Orbit
    Open
      Blowout Fracture: 21385–21395

The tabular section descriptions are then reviewed to assign the correct code.

80. C: As noted in the CPT guidelines regarding maternity care and delivery, antepartum care includes the initial prenatal history and physical, subsequent prenatal history and physicals, recording of weight, blood pressures, fetal heart tones, routine chemical urinalysis, monthly visits to 28 weeks, biweekly visits to 36 weeks, and weekly visits until delivery.

81. D: Code 81217 is assigned from the Gene Analysis Tier 1 Procedures category in the Pathology and Laboratory section. Using the CPT index, this can be found with the following:

Gene Analysis
  Analysis
    BRCA2: 81162–81164, 81167, 81212, 81216, 81217

The tabular section descriptions are then reviewed to assign the correct code.

82. D: Code 99401 is assigned from the Counseling Services: Risk Factor and Behavioral Change Modification category in the Evaluation and Management section. Using the CPT index, this can be found with the following:

Evaluation and Management Services
  Preventive: 99381–99429

The tabular section descriptions are then reviewed to assign the correct code. The instructional note states that issues such as healthy diet and exercise are included. Services may be provided separately to a new or established patient and may be performed by a physician or other qualified healthcare professional.

83. A: Code 99509 is assigned from the Home Visit by a Non-Physician Professional category in the Medicine section. Using the CPT index, this can be found with the following:

Activities of Daily Living
  In-home Assistance: 99509
  Training: 97535

The tabular section descriptions are then reviewed to assign the correct code. CPT code 97535 is incorrect because the code description does not limit the site of service to a home visit and includes training, whereas CPT code 99509 specifically states "home visit" for assistance with activities of daily living and personal care. It is important to code for the highest level of specificity while accurately covering the procedure as documented.

84. A: Code 99479 is assigned from the Initial Inpatient Neonatal Intensive Care and Other Services category in the Evaluation and Management section. Using the CPT index, this can be found with the following:

Evaluation and Management Services
  Neonatal
    Intensive Hospital Care: 99477–99480

The tabular section descriptions are then reviewed to assign the correct code.

85. D: Code 94762 is assigned from the Respiratory Services: Diagnostic and Therapeutic category in the Medicine section. Using the CPT index, this can be found with the following:

Oximetry
  Blood Oxygen Saturation Determination
    Noninvasive Ear or Pulse: 94760–94762

The tabular section descriptions are then reviewed to assign the correct code.

86. C: Code 90832 is assigned from the Psychotherapy Services category in the Medicine section. Using the CPT index, this can be found with the following:

Psychotherapy
  Individual Patient: 90832–908234, 90836–90838

The tabular section descriptions are then reviewed to assign the correct code. There is an instructional note at code 90863 to first code 90832, 90834, or 90837. The question states 30 minutes of psychotherapy, and no mention is made of an evaluation and management service; therefore, code 90863 for pharmacological management is assigned as a secondary CPT code.

87. A: Code 17110 is correct because *ablation* means the destruction of benign, premalignant, or malignant tissues by any method, which includes laser, electrosurgery, cryosurgery, and chemical treatment.

First, search the CPT index for the following:

Destruction
  Lesion
    Skin
      Benign: 17110, 17111

88. C: Code 62282 is assigned from the Spine and Spinal Cord, Injection, Drainage, or Aspiration category in the Nervous System chapter. Using the CPT index, this can be found with the following:

Injection
  Spinal Cord
    Neurolytic Agent: 62280–62282

The tabular section descriptions are then reviewed to assign the correct code.

89. B: Codes 57456 and 58110-59 are assigned from the Cervix Uteri, Endoscopy category in the Female Genital System chapter. CPT code 57456 describes a colposcopy with endocervical curettage. There is an instructional note with the conization procedure (code 57461) that it is not to be reported as an addition to code 57456. There is a separate instructional note stating that when an endometrial biopsy is performed in conjunction with a colposcopy, use code 58110. Refer to Appendix A for the definitions of CPT modifiers.

90. B: Code 67901-50 is assigned from the Repair (Brow Ptosis, Blepharoptosis) category in the Eye and Ocular Adnexa chapter. Using the CPT index, this can be found with the following:

Blepharoptosis
  Repair: 67901-67909

or

Frontalis Muscle Technique: 67901

Refer to CPT Appendix A for descriptions of the modifiers.

91. C: Code 74400 is assigned from the Urogenital category in the Radiology section. Using the CPT index, this can be found with the following:

Pyelogram: 74400

92. C: Code 32662 is assigned from the Thoracic Surgery: Video-Assisted category in the Respiratory System section. Using the CPT index, this can be found with the following:

Thoracoscopy
  Surgical
    With Excision of Mediastinal Cyst, Tumor, and/or Mass: 32662

93. A: The OIG-issued General Compliance Program Guidance recommends that small entities should conduct an audit at least once annually. Based on the audit results, the entity will be able to determine whether there are issues that it should address, including repayment of any overpayments that were discovered during the audit. The guidance does not require that an audit be performed by an outside entity, but it does suggest that outside assistance may be necessary to investigate, address, and resolve any compliance issues. It does require that exclusion lists be assessed, and it requires that any payments be returned for excluded participants of a federal health-care program, but it does not mention workers' compensation. Provider bonuses are not mentioned in the compliance guidance.

94. B: CPT instructions in the Repair-Closure category of the Integumentary section state that complex repairs include the debridement of wound edges for traumatic lacerations or avulsion injuries in addition to an intermediate repair. Code 13121 is for the complex repair of a wound (2.6–7.5 cm in size) to the scalp, arms, or legs.

95. A: Code 00142 is assigned from the Anesthesia for Eye Procedures category in the Anesthesia section. Using the CPT index, this can be found with the following:

Anesthesia
  Eye
    Lens Surgery: 00142

96. B: Code 62165 is assigned from the Skull, Meninges and Brain, Neuroendoscopy category in the Nervous System chapter. Using the CPT index, this can be found with the following:

Neuroendoscopy
    Intracranial: 62160–62165

The tabular section descriptions are then reviewed to assign the correct code.

97. D: First, search the ICD-10 index for the following:

Examination
    Pre-procedural
        Specified NEC: Z01.818
Fibroid
    Uterus: D25.9

Then, confirm the coding in the tabular list. It is important to note that the Z01.81 category includes encounters for radiological and imaging examination as part of a preprocedural examination. Chapter 21 guidance indicates which Z codes may only be a principal diagnosis, and that list includes the Z01 category. See Chapter 21 Guideline I.C.21.c.16 to review the entire list.

98. C: Code 88142 is assigned from the Pap Smears category in the Pathology and Laboratory section. Using the CPT index, this can be found with the following:

Cytopathology
    Cervical or Vaginal
        Thin Layer Prep: 88142, 88143, 88174, 88175

The tabular section descriptions are then reviewed to assign the correct code.

99. D: Codes 63047, 63048 are assigned from the Spine and Spinal Cord, Posterior Extradural Laminotomy or Laminectomy category in the Nervous System chapter. Using the CPT index, this can be found with the following:

Laminectomy
    For Decompression
        Lumbar: 0275T, 63005, 63012, 63017, 63047, 63048

The tabular section descriptions are then reviewed to assign the correct code. Decompression of the nerve roots will lead to the code assignment of 63047, which is either unilateral or bilateral. The add-on code 63048 is for each additional vertebral (lumbar) segment—in this case, for L2.

100. A: Code 74022 is assigned from the Abdomen category in the Radiology section. Using the CPT index, this can be found with the following:

Abdomen
    X-ray: 74018, 74019, 74021, 74022

The description of code 74022 states that the acute abdomen series includes a single chest view. The tabular section descriptions are then reviewed to assign the correct code.

CPC Practice Test #2

1. What is the correct CPT code assignment for the following scenario?

A 34-year-old female patient is seen in the operating room for partial distal gastrectomy with formation of an intestinal pouch. A vagotomy will also be performed in this session.

a. 43622, 43635
b. 43640, 43631-51
c. 43634, 43635
d. 43634, 43635-59

2. What is the correct CPT code assignment for the following scenario?

A 68-year-old patient presents for a transurethral resection of the prostate (TURP) procedure due to recurrent bladder outlet obstruction, secondary to prostate enlargement. This patient underwent a prior TURP procedure 14 years ago, so regrowth of obstructive tissue is suspected.

a. 52500
b. 52601, 52630-51
c. 52630
d. 52601

3. Fractures can be specified as open or closed and as displaced or nondisplaced. In cases of fractures that lack these designations, the ICD-10-CM codes should default to which of the following?

a. Open and displaced
b. Closed and displaced
c. Open and nondisplaced
d. Closed and nondisplaced

4. A new patient is seen at her residence for care. The encounter ran for 1 hour in total. A history was gathered, and an examination was performed. The patient has type 2 diabetes that she has managed long-term with diet and exercise. The patient is in good spirits today, and a low level of medical decision-making was required for this encounter. What CPT code should be used for this visit?

a. 99205
b. 99342
c. 99350
d. 99344

5. A 46-year-old patient is seen at the chiropractic clinic after a fall from a motorcycle, complaining of sharp pain in his lower back. At the time of the accident, no fractures were observed on x-ray. Today, the chiropractor will manipulate the patient's lower spine in the lower lumbar region as well as S1 (i.e., the first vertebra of the sacral region). What is the correct CPT code assignment for this visit?

a. 98940×2
b. 98940
c. 98943
d. 98925

6. A patient visits urgent care with fractures to both thumbs after falling from a horse. According to the ICD-10-CM guidelines in Section I.B., how should the diagnoses of these injuries be reported?

a. S62.5XXX
b. S62.501A, S62.502A
c. S62.50XA-50
d. S62-LT, -RT

7. A 22-year-old man will be receiving a right lung today after many months on the transplant list. The organ donor was pronounced dead on arrival at the hospital after a motorcycle accident and is confirmed as an organ donor. What is the correct CPT code assignment and sequencing for the cadaver pneumonectomy, allograft backbench preparation, and insertion of the lung into the recipient under cardiopulmonary bypass? (Note that each of these procedures is to be performed by a different surgeon on the same surgical team.)

a. 32852-RT
b. 32850, 32851-51
c. 32852, 32850-RT, 32855
d. 32850, 32855, 32852

8. Which of the following is true about billing for diagnostic thoracoscopy with a surgical thoracoscopy (i.e., video-assisted thoracoscopic surgery [VATS])?

a. Unbundling the diagnostic procedure from the VATS procedure may only be done if no anesthesia is used in either procedure.
b. Surgical thoracoscopy may be performed on a different day than the diagnostic thoracoscopy so that they can be billed as separate procedures.
c. VATS always includes diagnostic thoracoscopy.
d. Diagnostic thoracoscopy is a separate procedure and must be billed in addition to the VATS procedure.

9. When an acute condition and a chronic condition are documented with separate codes, which of the following is correct based on ICD-10-CM guidelines?

a. Report both codes in alphabetical order.
b. Report both codes in the sequence of oldest condition to newest condition.
c. Report both codes, with the acute code first.
d. Only code chronic conditions once, whether or not both acute and chronic codes are reported.

10. Diagnosis: mitral valve prolapse

A 33-year-old female patient is seen in the OR for insertion of a mitral valve ring due to prolapse of the mitral valve. The patient undergoes cardiopulmonary bypass for this procedure.

What is the correct CPT code assignment?

a. 33430
b. 33425, 33422
c. 33426
d. 33422, 33426-51

11. Diagnosis: radial fracture, right side

The patient is a 26-year-old male with a fractured radius. Upon physical examination in the office today and review of his prior radiographs taken here last week, the patient is directed to maintain use of his arm sling and full rest for the injured area, to the fullest extent possible (it is a dominant-side injury). The patient will come back in 2 weeks for new x-rays to be taken and for reassessment of his plan.

What is the correct CPT code assignment for this visit?

a. 99213
b. 99214
c. 99203
d. 99221

12. A patient will be treated for multiple areas of molluscum contagiosum on the penis. This will be a simple procedure using cryosurgery. What is the correct CPT code assignment?

a. 54065
b. 54056
c. 54050, 54065-51
d. 54115

13. What is the correct HCPCS Level II code for a nutritionally complete enteral formula for administration by feeding tube—including hydrolyzed proteins, fats, carbohydrates, vitamins, and minerals—that is NOT specified for pediatric use?

a. B4154
b. B4161
c. B4153
d. B4220

14. The axial skeleton includes which of the following bones?

a. Skull and other bones of the head, shoulders, rib cage, and arms
b. Shoulders, pelvis, arms, and legs
c. Shoulders, rib cage, pelvis, and spine
d. Skull and other bones of the head, rib cage, and spine

15. Pre- and postoperative diagnosis: intradural lesion of sacrum, right S2–S3

Procedure note:

Laminectomy with resection of intradural lesion, which extends to the post-S3 nerve root. Labs of resected lesion returned as negative for evidence of cancerous cells. May consult with the patient after recovery for future reconstructive procedure dependent upon mobility.

Which of the following choices is the correct CPT code for the procedure?

a. 63283
b. 63290×2
c. 63283, 63295
d. 63283×2

16. Which of the following would best fall under a HCPCS Level II code?

a. Radiation treatment management
b. A diagnostic colonoscopy
c. A malignant neoplasm
d. Advanced life support

17. A 49-year-old woman was seen in the OR for a modified radical mastectomy. Although the plan also included performing a dissection of her mammary nodes, only the mastectomy proved to be necessary. What is the correct CPT code assignment for anesthesia for the performed procedure?

a. 00400, 00406-59
b. 00404, 00402-59
c. 00406
d. 00404

18. A patient is seen in the OR for removal of a Bartholin's gland. This is a simple procedure that the patient tolerates well, and she is discharged later the same day. What is the correct CPT assignment for this procedure?

a. 56501
b. 56440
c. 56740
d. 56420

19. What are the three ways by which contrast material can be injected for radiology?

a. Intranasally, intravascularly, intrathecally
b. Intracranially, intrapleurally, intra-articularly
c. Intravascularly, intrathecally, intracranially
d. Intravascularly, intra-articularly, intrathecally

20. HCPCS Level II modifiers are appended to CPT procedural codes to add specificity for body parts including all of the following EXCEPT:

a. Coronary arteries (right, left, and branch)
b. Reduced services or increased services to either left or right laterality, but not both
c. Eyelids (right, left, upper, lower)
d. Fingers and toes (by laterality and by digit)

21. A patient receives percutaneous pleural drainage with catheter insertion, using ultrasound guidance. What is the correct CPT code assignment?

a. 32557, 75989-51
b. 32557
c. 32551
d. 32550, 32557-51

22. A 33-year-old male motorist is seen in the emergency department for injuries following an automobile accident. The physician suspects that the patient is drunk. What type(s) of tests may be performed to determine the presence or absence of alcohol in the patient's system and the amount of alcohol currently in his bloodstream?

a. A qualitative test to determine both whether there is alcohol in the patient's system and how much alcohol is in his bloodstream

b. A qualitative test to determine the presence or absence of alcohol in the patient's system, and a quantitative test to determine how much alcohol is in his bloodstream
c. A quantitative test to determine the presence or absence of alcohol in the patient's system, and a qualitative test to determine how much alcohol is in his bloodstream
d. A qualitative test to determine the presence or absence of alcohol in the patient's system, and a second qualitative test to determine how much alcohol is in his bloodstream

23. An 8-year-old boy is being treated in the emergency department for second-degree burns to the fronts of his legs and the tops of his feet. The burns were caused by a hot oil spill when the boy accidentally knocked a pot off the stove. Most of the burns were to his feet, and his legs were burned when the liquid splashed after the initial spill. His TBSA is 12%. His burns were debrided and dressed. What is the correct CPT code assignment?

a. 16030
b. 16020, 16025-51
c. 16030×2
d. 16035

24. A 26-year-old woman slipped on some ice and fell down her porch steps, twisting her right knee and falling directly on her kneecap. She is seen in her doctor's office to determine if she has a sprain or a tear. The physician also orders an x-ray to rule out fracture, and a complete scan is done directly in the office that day. The x-ray results show a hairline fracture to the patella. What is the correct CPT radiology code assignment for this visit, with the physician reading the x-ray scan and reporting on it?

a. 73564
b. 73564-26
c. 73580-26, 73565-50-51
d. 73560-RT, 73564-51-RT

25. When coding for sequelae, how should the residual condition and the cause of the condition be coded?

a. The residual condition only
b. The original illness or injury only
c. The residual condition, then the original illness or injury
d. The original illness or injury, then the residual condition

26. An elderly female patient is seen by her doctor to have her senile osteoporosis monitored. It is found that due to her osteoporosis, she now has osteoarthritis focused in both of her hip joints and her left shoulder. What is the correct ICD-10-CM code assignment?

a. M16.6, M19.212, M81.0
b. M16.7-RT, M16.7-LT, M19.21
c. M16.0, Q78.2
d. M81.0, M16.6, M19.212

27. A 17-year-old female patient arrives after a boating accident and is admitted by a hospitalist for observation. Another provider discharges her the following day. Which category and subcategory of E/M codes would be selected for the hospitalist's services?

a. Outpatient consultation
b. Initial hospital inpatient or observation care
c. Office visit, new patient
d. Preventive medicine, new patient

28. What HCPCS code is used for a 30 mg dose of Zemaira administered intravenously?

a. J0291
b. J0248×3
c. J0257×30
d. J0256×3

29. Which of the following is NOT a widely used method of tubal ligation, a female sterilization procedure?

a. Cauterize
b. Bands
c. Staple
d. Tie and cut

30. What is the correct CPT code assignment for the following encounter?

Pre- and postoperative diagnosis: splenorrhaphy
Procedure performed: complete splenectomy
Procedural notes: Under general anesthesia, the ruptured spleen was removed. The patient tolerated the procedure well and was awakened to return to the recovery suite.

a. 38100, 38102
b. 38120
c. 38102
d. 38100

31. An extracorporeal shock wave therapy (i.e., lithotripsy) procedure is performed on the right kidney of a 36-year-old woman. She also requires placement of a right ureteral stent. What is the correct CPT code assignment?

a. 52344-RT, 50590-51-RT
b. 50590-RT, 52341-51
c. 50947-RT, 50590-51-RT
d. 50590-RT, 52332-51-RT

32. Which of the following statements is NOT true regarding the liver?

a. It rids the body of ammonia, a toxic by-product of protein digestion.
b. It is the second-largest organ in the human body, after the skin.
c. It converts excess glucose into glycogen.
d. It is one of only three organs in the human body with the capability to self-regenerate.

33. A past patient is seen today for a comprehensive annual physical and pelvic examination, after not having a preventive appointment or other care for 6 years. She is 46 years old. Vital signs are taken, and her medical history and current medications are discussed. Physical, breast, and pelvic exams are performed and a Pap smear is collected. What is the correct CPT code assignment?

a. 99202
b. 99381
c. 99396
d. 99386

34. A 54-year-old male is seen in the OR for a ureterosigmoidostomy as part of a complete cystectomy procedure. External hypogastric and iliac lymph nodes of the pelvis will also be removed bilaterally. What is the correct CPT code assignment?

a. 51585
b. 51595
c. 51575
d. 51535, 51585-50

35. What CPT code assignment is reported for an extraoral incision and drainage of a cyst of the floor of the mouth in the masticator space?

a. 41018
b. 41009
c. 41000, 41018-51
d. 41015-50

36. What is the correct CPT code assignment for the following scenario?

A 46-year-old patient involved in a motor vehicle accident is seen in the emergency department with extensive injuries. One of his conditions is a diaphragmatic hernia that will be repaired in the OR once he is stabilized.

a. 39501
b. 39540
c. 39560, 39501-59
d. 39541, 39540-51

37. A 51-year-old male patient who has been awaiting a liver transplant received a call today that a match has become available. The patient's formal diagnosis is cirrhosis of the liver, nutritional. The patient has an extensive personal and family history of alcohol dependence, although he is now sober. What is the correct ICD-10-CM code assignment for this diagnosis?

a. K74.60, K70.30
b. K70.30, F10.20
c. F10.20, K70.30
d. K74.60, F10.10

38. In what care category is the time spent in treating a patient NOT considered in determining the level of medical decision-making and therefore in selecting the correct E/M code?

a. Interprofessional telehealth consultations
b. Counseling risk factor reduction
c. Emergency department services
d. Hospital observation care

39. What is the name of the sensory and motor nerve located in the skin of the lower abdomen, gluteal region, and portions of the abdominal muscles?

a. Saphenous nerve
b. Subcostal nerve
c. Pudendal nerve
d. Iliohypogastric nerve

40. What is the correct CPT code assignment for anesthesia services for a cleft palate repair?

a. 00102
b. 00172
c. 00170
d. 00176

41. Which of the following is NOT contained within the subcutaneous layers of skin?

a. Blood vessels
b. Keratin
c. Cutaneous nerves
d. Sweat glands

42. What is the correct CPT code assignment for a proximal subtotal pancreatectomy with total duodenectomy, partial gastrectomy, choledochoenterostomy, and gastrojejunostomy with pancreatojejunostomy?

a. 48145
b. 48150
c. 48001
d. 48160, 48152-51

43. A patient with chromosome abnormalities is seen by a cytopathologist and has a flow cytometry scheduled for interpretation. Twelve markers are to be reviewed. What is the correct CPT assignment?

a. 88187×6
b. 88188
c. 88199
d. 88184, 88185×11

44. A diaphragm resection and repair are done using a biologic mesh to reduce the formation of adhesions. Which procedure code should be reported?

a. 39501
b. 39560
c. 39561
d. 39599

45. A patient with diabetes is seen at their local clinic for the following immunizations: influenza, trivalent (IIV3) split virus, 0.25mL; and tetanus, diphtheria toxoids, and acellular pertussis (Tdap). Both immunizations were delivered intramuscularly. What are the correct CPT codes for this visit?

a. 90471, 90473
b. 90658, 90715
c. 90657, 90715, 90471, 90472
d. 90714, 90657, 90471×2

46. Which of the following roots refers to the common bile duct?

a. *Choledoch/o-*
b. *Chol/o-*
c. *Cholangi/o-*
d. *Cholecyst/o-*

47. A group education session is offered to four newly diagnosed adolescent type 1 diabetes patients along with their parents or caregivers. A registered dietitian meets with the group for 2 hours to go over diabetes management and lifestyle choices and hold a question-and-answer period. What is the correct CPT code assignment for this session?

a. 98961×4
b. 98961×2
c. 98960×4
d. 98968×4

48. A spiral fracture of the tibia is repaired by manipulation only, under anesthesia, without surgery. What is the correct description of this procedure?

a. Closed treatment of a comminuted fracture
b. Semiclosed treatment of a dislocation
c. Open treatment of a closed fracture
d. Closed treatment of a closed fracture

49. Evaluation and management (E/M) codes may report payable services within the global package, and they are appended with modifiers to denote this. Which of the following is NOT a global package E/M modifier?

a. -25: significant, separately identifiable E/M service by the same physician on the same day of the procedure or other service
b. -57: decision for surgery
c. -27: multiple outpatient hospital E/M encounters on the same date
d. -24: unrelated E/M service by the same physician during the postoperative period

50. The thoracic diaphragm enables respiration and speech and divides what two sections of the body from one another?

a. Abdomen and mediastinum
b. Lymphatic channels and mediastinum
c. Thoracic cavity and abdomen
d. Lungs and thoracic cavity

51. A cardiologist performs an atrial ablation and reconstruction procedure on a 58-year-old patient. At the end of the procedure, she performs a sternal closure using suture. What CPT code(s) should be reported?

a. 33255
b. 33255, 21750
c. 33255, 21750-78
d. 33255, 13160

52. What is the correct ICD-10-CM code assignment for a diagnosis of type 2 diabetes mellitus with diabetic chronic kidney disease (CKD) stage 3a?

a. E11.22, N18.31
b. E11.21, N18.30
c. E11.29, N18.3
d. E11.22, N18.4

53. Which of the following statements is NOT correct for bypass graft procedures?

a. Procurement of the vein for a saphenous vein graft procedure is included in the procedure codes that specify bypass graft.
b. Add-on code 35500 for harvest of an upper extremity vein should be added to certain bypass graft codes.
c. When reporting bypass graft code 35570 for a tibial-tibial graft, additional coding for vessel repairs should be used.
d. There is a single code that includes all procedural elements of an autogenous composite of three or more graft segments taken from distant sites.

54. What is the correct CPT code assignment for the following scenario?

A patient diagnosed with sarcoidosis of the lymph nodes undergoes a mediastinotomy. Under general anesthesia, an incision is made over the trachea in a standard linear fashion. Two very enlarged lymph nodes are discovered and extensively biopsied. All specimens are sent to pathology, and the patient is awakened and taken to recovery in stable condition.

a. 39220
b. 39402, 39000-51
c. 39010
d. 39000

55. A 7-year-old girl fell while hiking in the woods with her family. She fell onto her walking stick, which caused a deep, 2-cm-long laceration on the vestibule of her oral cavity. She is brought in by her parents and siblings, and a complex repair is performed in the office. She is sent home with treatment advice of rest and over-the-counter medication for any pain. What is the correct CPT code assignment for this procedure?

a. 40831
b. 40830
c. 40844
d. 40804, 40830-59

56. A 42-year-old male undergoes excision of the thymus gland. A partial removal is scheduled, but during the procedure it is decided that the entire thymus must be removed. The full thymectomy is performed via the transthoracic approach. What is the correct CPT code assignment?

a. 60521-22
b. 60522
c. 60520
d. 60521

57. What is the correct CPT code assignment for the following?

Pre- and postoperative diagnosis: Achilles tendon rupture, right side
Procedure performed: open repair of the right-side Achilles tendon
Procedural notes: Under general anesthesia, an incision was made longitudinally and near-complete rupture of the Achilles was observed. We repaired the rupture with debridement and by securing both ends of the tendon with wire and sutures.

a. 27650-RT
b. 27685-RT
c. 27654
d. 27650, 27652-51-RT

58. Which of the following statements is NOT true of the mediastinum?

a. It contains blood vessels and is located in the right upper abdominal quadrant.
b. It contains the thymus gland, which plays a role in immunity and autoimmunity.
c. It contains the heart, aorta, esophagus, and trachea.
d. It contains nerves.

59. A 30-year-old female patient is diagnosed with Hodgkin lymphoma. Bone marrow will be taken from a donor, her twin brother, to be transplanted into the patient as part of her treatment plan. What CPT code is reported for the harvesting of donor marrow from her brother?

a. 38222
b. 38220, 38230-51
c. 38230
d. 38232

60. CPT code assignment for anesthetic procedures considers the upper and lower abdomen to be separate regions. Each abdominal region contains both intraperitoneal and extraperitoneal organs. Which of the following statements is correct?

a. The stomach is an intraperitoneal organ of the lower abdomen.
b. The appendix is an extraperitoneal organ of the upper abdomen.
c. The spleen is an extraperitoneal organ of the upper abdomen.
d. The bladder is an extraperitoneal organ of the lower abdomen.

61. Which government agency is tasked with protecting the integrity of the Department of Health and Human Services' programs and their beneficiaries?

a. Office of Inspector General
b. Government Accountability Office
c. Department of Justice
d. American Medical Association

62. Which of the following terms is NOT a directional term related to anatomical positions for medical documentation?

a. Superficial
b. Inferial
c. Distal
d. Supine

63. According to the CPT instructions, under which of the following circumstances is a patient considered a new patient?

a. When a patient is under observation status at a hospital but is then transitioned to inpatient care
b. When a physician moves from one practice to another and a past long-term patient schedules an appointment at the physician's new location 1 year later
c. When a long-term patient schedules an appointment with a physician after not seeing the provider for 4 years
d. When a nurse practitioner rather than the physician sees a patient within the same practice

64. A patient is seen for preemployment screening as part of the hiring process at the local power plant. A comprehensive metabolic panel is ordered, along with a thyroid-stimulating hormone test, automated complete blood count, and automated differential white blood cell count. What is the correct CPT code assignment for these tests?

a. 80053, 85025, 85004, 84443
b. 80048, 80053
c. 80047
d. 80050

65. What is the correct CPT code assignment for the following scenario?

Pre- and postoperative diagnosis: dislocation, left elbow; fracture, proximal ulnar, left
Procedure performed: closed reduction of both ulnar fracture and elbow dislocation
Procedural notes: Under general anesthesia, we performed a reduction of the elbow, and it was noted as stable. We manipulated the ulna as well and were able to reduce it within the closed procedure. Patient to recover with use of long arm splint and over-the-counter pain medication as needed.

a. 24685-LT, 24605-51-LT
b. 24685, 24600
c. 24670-LT, 24605-51-LT
d. 24605-LT, 24670-59-LT

66. A 29-year-old patient has been on the waiting list for a kidney transplant. An appointment is made with a psychologist to assess whether the patient will be able to comply with recovery program requirements once a donor match is made. What is the correct CPT code assignment for a 1-hour session with this specialist?

a. 96158×2
b. 96158, 96159×2
c. 96156
d. 96160

67. A 24-year-old woman who has a 7-year personal history of eating disorders has an appointment at the clinic due to a recent rapid weight loss of 43 pounds. The patient claims to have behavior patterns of binge eating and then forcing herself to vomit. What is the correct diagnosis and code assignment for this visit?

a. F50.00, R63.4
b. F50.0X
c. F50.02
d. F50.2, F50.02

68. Which of the following is Figure I.C.15.a.1 in the ICD-10-CM guidelines?

a. Sepsis, severe sepsis, and septic shock
b. Adverse effect, poisoning, underdosing, and toxic effects
c. Conditions affecting pregnancy
d. Codes from Chapter 15 and sequencing priority

69. Psychiatric services, which may be reported with CPT codes 90791–90792 as well as E/M codes, include all of the following EXCEPT:

a. Clinical psychologists
b. Family and marriage counselors
c. Clinical social workers
d. Physicians specializing in psychiatry

70. Under CPT surgery guidelines, a global surgery status indicator classifies minor or major surgery based on relative value unit calculations. Which of the following is NOT a correct status indicator?

a. MMM for maternity codes, which are outside the usual global concept
b. 000 for outpatient vasectomies or intrauterine device insertions
c. 010 for minor procedures with a 10-day postoperative period
d. 090 for major procedures with a 90-day postoperative period

71. A patient with a personal history of lymphoma now has a mass in his right cervical lymph node. A node excisional biopsy beneath the muscle layers is performed because it is suspected that the lymphoma may be recurring. What is the correct CPT code assignment for this procedure?

a. 38500, 38555-51
b. 38510
c. 38520
d. 38500, 38510-51

72. Preparation for a surgical procedure includes ordering two units of frozen blood. What is the correct CPT code assignment for the preparation of the frozen blood, including freezing and thawing?

a. 86930×2, 86931-59×2
b. 86930, 86931
c. 86932×2
d. 86985-26

73. Assign the appropriate procedure and diagnosis codes for a biopsy of a posterior mediastinal mass that was obtained through an incision at the base of the neck.

a. 39000, D38.3
b. 39401, D49.89
c. 39000, R22.2
d. 39401, R22.1

74. A 70-year-old patient is discharged from the hospital after an emergency appendectomy. Due to existing mobility issues, the patient will need help for the next 10 days or so with personal care and daily activities. A home health agency is contacted by the physician's office for this service. What is the correct CPT code assignment for the home health service?

a. 99507
b. 99509
c. 99600
d. 99509×10, 99600×10

75. For the last week, an 85-year-old man with a cerebrospinal fluid shunt system has been having complications with the shunt not draining properly. The system was originally placed 3 weeks ago. Due to the buildup of excess cerebrospinal fluid, the surgeon sees the patient in the OR to remove the shunt system. For now, due to the patient's advanced age and other compounding health problems, there will be a recovery period before deciding whether to replace the shunt system. The surgeon who placed the system originally also performs its removal. What CPT code is reported?

a. 62258
b. 62252-78
c. 62256-78
d. 62256

76. A 25-year-old patient presents for excision of a benign lesion on the right side of his forehead, near the temple. The lesion measures 1.4 cm. The area is marked for excision with gross normal margins of 3–5 mm. What is the correct CPT code assignment for this procedure?

a. 11442-22
b. 11422
c. 11442
d. 11312

77. A 34-year-old patient with severe systemic disease is seen for a tubal ligation 6 months after the birth of her third child. What is the correct CPT code and physical status modifier for the anesthesia for this visit?

a. 00846-P2
b. 00921-P3
c. 00851-P3
d. 00851-P4

78. What is the correct CPT code assignment for the following?

Pre- and postoperative diagnosis: fracture, proximal tibia, left; dislocation, left patella.
Procedure performed: open reduction of tibial fracture, closed manipulation of patella dislocation.
Procedural notes: The patient was placed under general anesthesia in the OR. First, a closed reduction of the patellar dislocation was performed successfully, resulting in stability around the kneecap. Next, we manipulated the tibia, but we were unable to reduce it within the closed procedure. An incision was then made, and open reduction was performed on the fracture. After closing the incision, the patient was awakened from anesthesia and sent to recovery in stable condition.

a. 27535-LT, 27562-51-LT
b. 27562-51, 27535-22
c. 27524-LT, 27530-LT
d. 27530-LT, 27552-51-LT

79. What code assignment is reported for the following scenario?

In order to formally diagnose a patient experiencing ongoing problems with breathing, a sinusoscopy via puncture into the sphenoid sinus is performed during an endoscopic nasal procedure.

a. 31235-50
b. 31233
c. 31235
d. 31231, 31230

80. According to CPT instructions, when would code 49320 for peritoneoscopy (i.e., diagnostic laparoscopy) be reported?

a. Never, because a diagnostic laparoscopy is always included in surgical laparoscopy
b. In order to report a separate procedure code for diagnostic laparoscopy under certain circumstances
c. If a surgical laparoscopy is scheduled, but due to an anesthesia allergy, only a diagnostic procedure is performed
d. Always, because the peritoneoscopy should be unbundled from the surgical procedure

81. A young man presents to the ED with a sports injury to his clavicle. He collided with another player on the football field this morning when they both dove for a catch. The patient reports having heard a popping sound upon impact, followed by sharp pain when he hit the ground. The left collarbone area is inflamed and painful. What CPT code(s) should be reported by the radiologist performing x-rays of this area?

a. 73000
b. 73000-26
c. 73020-26-LT
d. 73000, 73020-59

82. A 66-year-old male comes to see his primary care physician, and during this appointment they discuss removal of his multiple skin tags that have been increasingly bothering him. After examining the patient's skin, the provider removes 23 skin tags across his shoulders, neck, and upper back. The provider uses a combination of the scissoring technique and ligature strangulation. What is the correct CPT code assignment for this visit?

a. 11200, 11201
b. 11200×23
c. 11305×23
d. 11200×15, 11201-51×8

83. What are the two layers of the serous pericardium?

a. Visceral and parietal
b. Fibrous and visceral
c. Parietal and vascular
d. Vascular and fibrous

84. A patient is seen for excision of approximately half of the left thyroid lobe, in addition to excision of the isthmus. What is the correct CPT code assignment?

a. 60210
b. 60212-LT
c. 60220, 60210-51
d. 60100

85. A patient is seen for urinalysis as part of a routine exam and workup. The physician is particularly interested in the patient's glucose, pH, and bilirubin levels. What is the correct CPT code assignment for this dipstick urinalysis if it is automated, without microscopy?

a. 81002, 81050-59
b. 81003
c. 81001, 81000-51
d. 81015

86. When a radiologist performs a procedure, what code modifier(s) are reported for the professional component and the technical component of the procedure?

a. Either -26 for the professional component or -TC for the technical component, but not both
b. Both -26 for the professional component and -TC for the technical component
c. Modifier -26 only because the professional component includes the technical component
d. No modifiers because the professional and technical components are both included in radiology procedure codes

87. A 40-year-old male is seen in the oncology department for radiation. He has appointments in the morning and in the afternoon for 3 days. This totals six fractions of radiation. What is the correct CPT code assignment for this radiation series?

a. 77431×3
b. 77427, 77431-51
c. 77427
d. 77469×6

88. Which of the following is NOT correct for ICD-10-CM coding of pressure ulcers by stage?

a. Stage 1: persistent focal edema
b. Stage 2: partial-thickness skin loss involving the epidermis, dermis, or both
c. Stage 3: full-thickness skin loss involving damage or necrosis of subcutaneous tissue
d. Stage 4: necrosis of soft tissue extending to underlying muscle or tendon, but not to the depth of the bone

89. A 49-year-old male undergoes cardiac catheterization in the cath lab. The right femoral artery is punctured for angiography, and then the catheter is placed in the aortic arch using fluoroscopy. What is the correct CPT code assignment?

a. 36246
b. 36221
c. 36200
d. 36215, 36218

90. An adolescent patient is seen for a radiological procedure following a motor vehicle accident the day before. His carotid artery sustained a small puncture and, although he is stable, the extent of the puncture is not yet known. What is the correct CPT code assignment for the anesthesia for this procedure?

a. 01925
b. 01916
c. 01916, 01924-59
d. 01922, 01924-590

91. CPT code modifiers -25 and -59 are both used to indicate significant, separately identifiable services performed on the same day as a primary service. Which of the following statements correctly describes when to use these modifiers?

a. Modifier -25 is used for E/M codes and -59 is used for all other codes.
b. Modifier -59 is used for surgery codes and -25 is used for all other codes.
c. Modifier -25 is used for E/M codes and -59 is used for surgery codes.
d. Modifier -25 is used for pathology and laboratory procedure codes and -59 is used for all other codes.

92. A 73-year-old man is seen for an upper abdominal surgery, a partial hepatectomy, without which he is not expected to survive. What is the correct CPT code assignment for the anesthesia for this procedure, including the physical status modifier for the patient, for this case?

a. 00792-P5
b. 00792-P4
c. 00790, 00792-59-P3
d. 00796-P6

93. Which of the following pairs of diagnoses may be coded as having a cause-and-effect relationship, even if not documented as such?

a. Hypertension and CKD
b. CKD and Lyme disease
c. Disease of the mastoid process and heart disease
d. Diabetes and angina

94. A woman in remission from breast cancer presents for intradermal tattooing of both areolae after breast reconstruction. For the right and left breasts, the areas for tattoo placement are $10.75\ cm^2$ and $11.25\ cm^2$, respectively. What is the correct CPT code assignment for this procedure?

a. 11921×2
b. 11921, 11922-51
c. 11920, 11922
d. 11921, 11922

95. A convenience store robbery has resulted in a 24-year-old male sustaining a fatal gunshot wound. He was brought to the ED earlier in critical condition and later succumbed to his injury and was pronounced deceased. What CPT code assignment is correct for the autopsy that must be performed to gather evidence for the police investigation?

a. 88040
b. 88000
c. 88040-90
d. 88099, 88020-59

96. A compliance plan is a written process for coding and submitting accurate claims. According to AAPC, the benefits of a compliance plan could include all of the following EXCEPT:

a. Faster, more accurate payment of claims
b. Fewer billing mistakes
c. Increased likelihood of higher revenue
d. Diminished chances of a payer audit

97. A patient receives a diagnostic computed tomography (CT) colonography, with and without contrast. What is the correct CPT code assignment?

a. 74280
b. 74263×2
c. 74261, 74262-59
d. 74262

98. What is the correct CPT code assignment for the following scenario?

Postoperative diagnosis: sterilization
Procedure performed: laparoscopic tubal ligation via bilateral application of oviduct bands
Procedural notes: Under general anesthesia, the right tube was ligated using the oviduct band. The same was then performed on the left tube. The patient was awakened from anesthesia and taken to the recovery room.

a. 58671-50
b. 58671
c. 58720
d. 58679

99. Under HIPAA regulations, which of the following is a policy requirement for "minimum necessary" access to protected health information?

a. Only the patient may have access.
b. Anyone employed at a provider's office may have access.
c. Only the treating physician may have access.
d. Access is provided only to those whose jobs require it.

100. According to the ICD-10-CM coding guidelines, which of the following is the correct sequence of steps in locating an ICD-10-CM code?

a. Locate the term in the alphabetic index, and then verify the code in the tabular list.
b. If the chart specifies poisoning or drug use, code only with the table of drugs and chemicals.
c. Locate the code in the tabular list, and then verify it in the alphabetic index.
d. If the chart specifies cancer or other tumors, code only with the table of neoplasms.

Answer Key and Explanations for Test #2

1. C: In the CPT index, look for Gastrectomy/Partial. Code 43634 is for the procedure with the specified intestinal pouch formation. Code 43635 is also needed for the vagotomy procedure, and since it is an add-on code, no modifier is needed. Code 43622 is for total gastrectomy, not partial; 43640 is for a separate vagotomy; and 43631 does not include the formation of the pouch.

2. C: In the CPT index, look for TURP. Only codes 52601 and 52630 are listed; code 52601 is for an initial procedure, so the correct single-code selection is 52630 for residual/regrowth of tissue. Code 52500 is for a transurethral resection, but of the bladder neck, not the prostate.

3. B: An undesignated fracture should be coded as closed and displaced in the absence of further documentation. ICD-10-CM Guideline I.C.19.c and Figure I.C.19.c give further instructions on proper coding and sequencing of traumatic fractures.

4. D: CPT guidelines on determining the level of evaluation and management services state that the greater of the two factors of time and medical decision-making (MDM) must be used for code selection. Code 99344 covers the 60 minutes for this encounter, which is the greater of the two factors in this case.

Code 99205 represents the correct time level (60 minutes), but it is for a new patient seen in a clinic, not at home. Code 99342 is for the correct MDM level (low), but according to the CPT guidelines, we must code for 60 minutes in this case. Code 99350 is correct for MDM and for a patient seen at home, but it specifies an established patient.

5. B: In the CPT Index, find Manipulation/Chiropractic. Of the code range given, 98940 describes the manipulation of one to two spinal regions, which is correct for lumbar and sacral manipulation. 98943 is for regions outside the spine, and 98925 is for an osteopathic treatment rather than a chiropractic one.

6. B: In the ICD-10-CM alphabetic index, look for Fracture, Traumatic/Thumb. Code S62.50 is given. Next, verify this code in the tabular list. Since no further details are given, use codes S62.501A and S62.502A for the initial encounter, traumatic fracture of the right and left thumbs respectively. This follows the guidelines in section I.B.13 regarding laterality, and it codes the encounter to the highest specificity using seven characters.

Modifiers -50, -LT, and -RT are for use with CPT procedural codes, not ICD-10-CM diagnosis codes.

7. D: In the CPT index, first look up Donor Procedures/Lung Excision, followed by Transplantation/Lung. The correct codes and sequencing are 32850 for cadaver lung removal, 32855 for unilateral backbench preparation, and 32852 for single lung transplant under bypass. A modifier for multiple procedures (-51) is not needed since each surgeon performed a procedure in series with the others and will each bill their service separately.

8. C: Diagnostic thoracoscopy is bundled into the surgical VATS procedure. Per CPT guidelines, diagnostic thoracoscopy cannot be billed separately during the same surgical session. Purposefully separating the procedures into different days in order to bill them separately constitutes billing fraud and could potentially be investigated.

9. C: Both acute and chronic codes should be reported, with the acute condition being sequenced first. Alphabetical order and sequencing codes from oldest to newest are not part of the ICD-10-CM guidelines. Chronic conditions that are treated on an ongoing basis may be coded as many times as required for proper care of the patient within the care plan.

10. C: In the CPT index, find Repair/Heart/Mitral Valve. Code 33426 for valvuloplasty is correct because it includes both the prosthetic ring and the bypass. Code 33430 is for a full mitral valve replacement, and this note specifies a repair with the prosthetic ring; 33425 is the correct procedure, but it does not include insertion of the prosthetic ring; and 33422 is for valvotomy, not valvuloplasty. Separate coding for the bypass is not needed here, since it is included in the stand-alone code 33426.

11. A: Since the patient has been seen in the past, he is an established patient. Codes for outpatient visits for established patients are evaluation and management (E/M) codes 99211–99215. To choose the appropriate medical decision-making (MDM) level and therefore the correct code, consider the patient's number and complexity of problems: one, which corresponds to low MDM. Next, consider the complexity of the data to be analyzed: one x-ray, which corresponds to minimal MDM. Next, consider the risk level: low, for sling care, which corresponds to low MDM. The correct code choice for outpatient care, established patient, low-level MDM is 99213.

Code 99214 would be for a moderate level of MDM; 99203 would be for a new patient visit; and 99221 would be for hospital (inpatient or observation) care, not outpatient care.

12. B: In the CPT index, codes 54050–54065 are for Destruction of Lesions of the Penis. The correct code for cryosurgical removal of molluscum contagiosum is 54056, while 54065 is for an extensive procedure, 54050 is for chemical means of removal, and 54115 is for removal of a foreign body.

13. C: In the HCPCS Level II index, find Enteral Nutrition/Formula/Hydrolyzed Proteins. The code given is B4153. There are many other options for both enteral and parenteral nutrition, but none are to the correct specificity: code B4154 does not include the hydrolyzed proteins, B4161 is specified for pediatric use, and B4220 is for the daily premixed nutrition supply kit.

14. D: The axial skeleton consists of the skull and other bones of the head, along with the rib cage and spine. The appendicular skeleton consists of the shoulders, pelvis, arms, and legs.

15. A: In the CPT index, locate Laminectomy/for Excision/Intraspinal Lesion/Neoplasm. Code 63283, laminectomy for intradural, sacral, is correct.

Code 63290 is for any level of lesion excision, but this code is not to the highest specificity since the note specifies a sacral lesion. Add-on code 63295 is not needed because the reconstructive procedure is only mentioned in the note as a potential post-recovery treatment. Code 63283 only needs to be specified once because only one intradural space is treated.

16. D: A HCPCS Level II code describes medical devices, supplies, medication, and/or other services that a provider and/or entity used during a service provided to a patient. Advanced life support (ALS) fits this description because it is a set of life-saving protocols administered in transit. Radiation treatment management and a diagnostic colonoscopy are reported by HCPCS Level I codes, otherwise known as CPT codes. If the patient was asymptomatic and the colonoscopy was for screening purposes only, a HCPCS Level II code could be assigned. However, a diagnostic procedure implies that there is a past medical/family history that puts the patient at risk and/or symptoms that warrant the procedure. A malignant neoplasm is reported with an ICD-10-CM code because it is a diagnosis.

17. D: In the CPT index, look for Anesthesia/Breast. The correct option for anesthesia for mastectomy only without mammary node dissection is 00404. Only this code is needed since only the mastectomy was performed. Code 00406 would be correct if the node dissection had also been performed; 00400 is for an unspecified procedure of the thorax; and 00402 is for breast reconstruction, which is often performed for patients undergoing mastectomy but is not specified in this procedural note.

18. C: In the CPT index, find Excision/Bartholin's Gland. Code 56740 is given. Code 56440 does cover this gland, but is a marsupialization procedure; 56420 is for treatment of an abscess; and 56501 is for treatment of a lesion of the vulva, not the Bartholin's gland.

19. D: The three ways that contrast material can be injected for radiology are intravascularly (via a vein or artery), intra-articularly (via a joint), and intrathecally (via a sheath, or within the subarachnoid space or cerebrospinal fluid). Contrast material may also be administered orally or rectally.

20. B: CPT-coded procedures performed on eyelids, fingers, toes, and coronary arteries are required to be appended with HCPCS Level II modifiers. These modifiers add greater specificity to show which part of the anatomy was treated. Modifiers for reduced services or increased services, however, are Level I modifiers and are not assigned based on laterality.

21. B: The stand-alone code for this procedure is 32557, and the ultrasound code 75989 is mentioned in the parenthetical notes below the drainage codes as "Do Not Use." Code 32550 is for a catheter with a cuff, which is not specified in the note, and code 32551 is for an open procedure, but this is a closed procedure using imaging.

22. B: A qualitative test is used determine the presence or absence of a substance. A quantitative test is used to determine how much of the substance is present. Note that a quantitative test can indicate presence/absence because a result of 0 means that the substance is not present. However, quantitative tests may be relatively slow, difficult, and/or expensive to perform, so a qualitative test may be performed first to determine if the quantitative test is necessary.

23. A: A second-degree burn is a partial-thickness burn. In the CPT index, look up Burns/Debridement, which gives the code range 16000–16036. With the patient's total body surface area (TBSA) of 12%, the correct code is 16030. It is reported only once even though two extremities were treated. Codes 16020 and 16025 are incorrect because the TBSA is calculated at 12%; 16035 is for an escharotomy, not a debridement.

24. A: In the CPT index, find X-ray/Knee. Code range 73560–73580 is given. Code 73564, "Radiologic examination, knee; complete, four or more views" is the correct choice. Because the physician read the report on a scan taken with his own x-ray equipment in his office, no modifier is needed for either a technical or professional component.

Code 73580 is for arthrography of the knee; 73565 is for a bilateral knee x-ray; 73560 is for a limited one- or two-view x-ray of the knee, and this procedure is noted as a complete (four-view) scan.

25. C: When coding sequelae, first code the residual condition. Next, code the original illness or injury that led to the sequelae as secondary.

26. A: The patient's osteoarthritis is considered secondary since it was caused by her osteoporosis. In the ICD-10-CM alphabetic index, look for Osteoarthritis/Secondary/Hip/Bilateral. Code M16.6 is given. Verify this code in the tabular list.

Next, look for Osteoarthritis/Secondary/Shoulder. Code M19.21 is given. Upon verification of this code in the tabular list, a sixth character is shown as required. Choose code M19.212 for the left shoulder.

Since the patient's secondary localized osteoarthritis is due to her osteoporosis, the osteoporosis should also be coded. Return to the alphabetic index and find Osteoporosis/Senile, which refers you to Osteoporosis/Age-related. Code M81.0 is given and should be verified in the tabular list.

Code M16.7 for unilateral osteoarthritis of the hip should not be used with -RT and -LT CPT modifiers; M19.21 is an incorrect code because it does not have the required sixth character for laterality (specified or unspecified); M16.0 is for osteoarthritis as a primary condition, not secondary; and M81.0 as the first-sequenced diagnosis code is incorrect because, although it is primary osteoporosis, it is not the primary diagnosis for this visit. The secondary osteoarthritis is the primary diagnosis for this visit. Code Q78.2 is a diagnosis code for osteosclerosis, a condition unrelated to this visit.

27. B: The patient is seen directly after the accident, so this is considered an initial visit. Since she is treated at a hospital, "Initial hospital inpatient" is the correct choice of E/M category and subcategory. An outpatient consultation, office visit, and preventive medicine visit would not apply since she is being treated in a hospital for injuries sustained in an accident.

28. D: In the HCPCS table of drugs, look up Zemaira. This drug is an alpha 1 proteinase inhibitor. The route of delivery is shown as intravenous, and the code for 10 mg is J0256; the correct code choice is therefore J0256×3. Code J0257 is also for an alpha-1 proteinase inhibitor, but it is only specified for the brand name Glassia, not Zemaira. Code J0291 is for the drug Zemdri, and J0248 is for Veklury.

29. C: Tubal ligation has a 99% success rate of preventing pregnancy. It is most frequently performed via cautery, bands, or tie and cut methods. Staples are not used in this procedure.

30. D: In the CPT index, look for Excision/Spleen. The correct code for total splenectomy is 38100. Code 38102 is an add-on code only; 38120 is for a laparoscopic procedure, which is not specified in the encounter notes.

31. D: In the CPT index, look up Extracorporeal Shock Wave Therapy/Lithotripsy and find code 50590. Modifier -RT specifies that the procedure is performed on the right kidney. Next, look up Insertion/Stent/Ureteral. Of the given code options 50947 and 52332, 50947 falls under laparoscopic procedures. Code 52332 is correct for insertion of an indwelling stent, with modifiers -51 and -RT to show that multiple procedures were performed and laterality, respectively. Code 50590 is listed first because it has more relative value units. Codes 52341 and 52344 are incorrect because neither includes the stent placement.

32. D: The liver does have the capability to self-regenerate; however, it is the only organ in the human body with this ability. The liver does rid the body of ammonia, is the second-largest organ, and does convert excess glucose into glycogen.

33. D: The patient is considered new because more than 3 years have passed since she was last seen. She is no longer an established patient. In the CPT index, look for Preventive

Care/Comprehensive/New Patient. Code range 99381–99387 is given. For this 46-year-old patient, code 99386 is the correct choice.

Code 99202 is for a new patient being seen in the office for a reason other than preventive care, 99381 is specific to patients younger than 1 year of age, and 99396 is for an established patient.

34. A: In the CPT index, find Cystectomy/Complete/with Bilateral Pelvic Lymphadenectomy. Of the code range 51575–51595 given, 51585 is for accompanying ureterosigmoidostomy. Codes 51575 and 51595 do not include the ureterosigmoidostomy; 51535 does not include the lymphadenectomy. Since code 51585 specifies bilateral removal, modifier -50 is not used.

35. A: In the CPT index, look for Drainage/Cyst/Mouth/Masticator Space. Codes 41009 and 41018 are the given options; select 41018 for extraoral. Code 41009 is for an intraoral procedure; 41000 is for the lingual space; 41015 is for the sublingual space, and modifier -50 for bilaterality is not needed.

36. B: Code 39540 is for repair of a traumatic acute hernia of the diaphragm, such as in a patient involved in a motor vehicle accident. Code 39501 is for laceration repair, 39541 is for a chronic hernia, and 39560 is for resection of the diaphragm.

37. B: In the ICD-10-CM alphabetic index, find Cirrhosis/Nutritional/Alcoholic. Code K70.30 is given. Verification in the tabular list shows that this is the correct code assignment for cirrhosis without ascites. Under the header code K70, an instruction is given to use an additional code to identify alcohol abuse and dependence F10.-. Beginning again with the alphabetic index, find Dependence/Alcohol, which refers to code F10.20. Verify this code as well by looking it up in the tabular list.

Code K74.60 is for cirrhosis but does not include any higher specificity; F10.10 is for nondependent alcohol abuse. The coding instruction to "use additional code" in section K70 of the tabular list shows that the correct coding sequence is to first code the cirrhosis, then code the alcohol dependence.

38. C: According to the CPT guidelines for E/M services, "Time is not a descriptive component for the emergency department levels of E/M services because emergency department services are typically provided on a variable intensity basis, often involving multiple encounters with several patients over an extended period of time."

Other categories, including interprofessional telehealth consultations, counseling risk factor reduction, and hospital observation, all include time as a component of MDM for code selection.

39. D: The iliohypogastric nerve is a sensory and motor nerve located in the skin of the lower abdomen, gluteal region, and portions of the abdominal muscles. The saphenous nerve is only sensory, not motor, and is located in the knee joint, patella, and the skin of the leg and foot. The subcostal nerve is a sensory and motor nerve that runs along the twelfth rib to the abdominal wall. The pudendal nerve is a sensory and motor nerve that is located in the pelvic region.

40. B: A cleft palate procedure is an intraoral procedure. In the CPT index, find Anesthesia/Intraoral Procedures. Code range 00170–00176 is given. The correct code choice is 00172. Code 00102 is for repair of a cleft lip, not cleft palate; 00170 is for an unspecified intraoral procedure, which is not specific enough; and 00176, radical surgery, is for a more invasive intraoral procedure than the one specified.

41. B: Keratin is contained within the epidermis, the top layer of skin. Blood vessels, the cutaneous nerves, and sweat glands are all contained within the subcutaneous skin layers.

42. B: In the CPT index, look for Pancreas/Excision/Partial. Code 48150 is for pancreatectomy, proximal subtotal with total duodenectomy; partial gastrectomy; choledochoenterostomy; and gastrojejunostomy (i.e., Whipple-type procedure) with pancreatojejunostomy. Code 48145 is for a distal procedure, not proximal; 48001 is for incision only, not excision; 48160 includes a transplant; and 48152 does not include pancreatojejunostomy.

43. B: In the CPT index, find Flow Cytometry. Of the code options given, code 88188 for 9–15 markers is the correct choice for the patient's 12 markers. Codes 88184 and 88185 are for cell surface, cytoplasmic, or nuclear markers, which are not specified in this case. Code 88187 is for 2–8 markers. Code 88199 is for an unlisted cytopathology procedure. Although not many details are given for coding this procedure, we do know that it is a flow cytometry order and must be coded as such.

44. C: A diaphragm resection is reported with CPT codes 39560-39561. The use of a biologic mesh makes the repair complex (code 39561), whereas a simple repair (code 39560) would implement only internal sutures.

45. C: In the CPT index, first find Vaccines and Toxoids/Influenza/for Intramuscular Use. Code 90657 is correct for the 0.25 mL dosage. Next, look for Vaccines and Toxoids/Tdap, and use code 90715. Codes 90471 and 90472 are also needed, as instructed by the guidelines, and they are the correct choices for intramuscular delivery. Code 90473 is for intranasal or oral delivery. Code 90714 is not the correct tetanus combination. Code 90658 is not the correct influenza vaccine dosage.

46. A: *Choledoch/o-* refers to the common bile ducts. *Chol/o-* refers to the bile or gall. *Cholangi/o-* refers to the bile ducts. *Cholecyst/o-* refers to the gallbladder.

47. A: In the CPT index, find Special Services/Group Education/Self-Management. This is considered special services because the registered dietician is the nonphysician healthcare professional providing the session. Code 98961 is the correct selection for a group size of four patients for up to 30 minutes, so a multiplier of 4 is used to account for the total of 2 hours. Code 98960 is the code for an individual session, and 98968 is for this type of session when offered by telephone.

48. D: A spiral fracture is a type of closed fracture, and nonsurgical manipulation of a fracture is a closed procedure.

49. C: Modifier -27 for multiple outpatient hospital E/M encounters occurring on the same date is not appended to E/M codes for services within a global package. Modifiers -24, -25, and -57 are all appended to E/M codes for services within a global package.

50. C: The thoracic diaphragm divides the thoracic cavity from the abdomen. The lymphatic channels, mediastinum, and lungs lie close to the diaphragm and work in conjunction with it.

51. A: The procedure is reported using CPT code 33255. A sternal closure is considered integral to this and any other open cardiac procedure when a sternal approach is used as the method of exposure, so the closure is not reported separately. If a sternal closure were performed as the only procedure to repair an injury, the closure would then be reported. CPT code 21750 is used for a sternal closure performed as a standalone procedure, with modifier -58 for a planned secondary procedure (such as an intentionally delayed closure) or modifier -78 for an unplanned secondary procedure. CPT code 13160 is used for complex closure of a wound, such as a surgical incision that has come apart or become infected.

52. A: ICD-10-CM **c**odes in the range of E11.2 are used to indicate type 2 diabetes mellitus with kidney complications. Code E11.22 specifies type 2 diabetes with diabetic chronic kidney disease (CKD). Code 11.21 is used for type 2 diabetes with diabetic nephropathy, which is a different type of kidney disease. Code E11.29 is used for type 2 diabetes with other diabetic kidney complication, which is incorrect because there is a code that specifies CKD.

An instructional note under E11.22 states that an additional code is used for the CKD stage. Codes N18.1–N18.6 specify these stages. Code 18.31 is used for CKD stage 3a. Codes 18.3 and 18.30 are correct for CKD stage 3, but the substage (3a) is not specified. Code N18.4 is used for stage 4 CKD.

53. C: In the CPT notes for bypass grafts, there are many guidelines and instructions. Code 35570 includes parenthetical notes stating that it should not be coded in conjunction with 35256 or 35286, both of which are for vessel repairs.

Saphenous vein procurement is included in the bypass code. Add-on code 35500 should be used for certain graft codes, such as 35510 for a carotid-brachial graft. Code 35683 is mentioned in the notes as being used for an autogenous composite of three or more segments.

54. D: Under Mediastinum in the CPT index, there are several options for biopsy. Code 39000 is the correct code because it specifies the cervical approach for the incision. Code 39010 is for the transthoracic approach; 39220 is for resection of a tumor, not a lymph node; and 39402 is for endoscopic procedures.

55. A: Look in the CPT Index for the following:

Repair
  Mouth
    Vestibule of

The code range 40830–40835 is given. Although the laceration is 2 cm in length, a complex repair is specified due to the depth of the injury. Code 40831 is the correct choice. Code 40830 is for lacerations 2.5 cm in length or less, but since this is a complex repair, code 40831 should be used regardless of the laceration measurement. Code 40844 is for vestibuloplasty of the entire arch of the oral cavity. Code 40804 is for removal of a foreign body, and the note does not specify that this was necessary.

56. D: In the CPT index, find Thymectomy/Transthoracic Approach. Code 60521 is the correct choice, and modifier -22 for increased procedural services is not needed because the code includes either partial or total removal of the gland. Code 60520 is for the same procedure but via a transcervical approach; 60522 includes radical dissection of the mediastinum, which is not specified in the surgeon's notes.

57. A: In the CPT index, look for Repair/Ankle/Tendon. This is a primary repair with no graft specified; therefore, 27650 with laterality modifier -RT is the correct code. Code 27685 is for a lengthening or shortening procedure, which is not specified in the procedural note.

58. A: Although the mediastinum does contain blood vessels, it is located between the lungs, not in the abdomen. The mediastinum also contains the thymus gland, heart, aorta, esophagus, trachea, and nerves.

59. C: In the CPT index, find Bone Marrow/Harvesting. Because it is harvested from a donor (allogeneic), code 38230 is the correct selection. Codes 38220 and 38222 are for diagnostic procedures, and 38232 is for harvesting the patient's own bone marrow (autologous).

60. D: The upper and lower abdomen anesthesia code ranges both include procedures on intraperitoneal and extraperitoneal organs. The bladder is in the lower abdomen and is an extraperitoneal organ. Upper abdominal organs are either intraperitoneal (stomach, liver, jejunum, and ascending and transverse colon) or extraperitoneal (kidneys, adrenal glands, and lower esophagus). Lower abdominal organs are also either intraperitoneal (appendix, cecum, ileum, and sigmoid colon) or extraperitoneal (ureters and bladder).

61. A: The Office of Inspector General offers compliance program guidance that forms the basis for provider practice compliance plans and has been doing so since the program was first published in October 2000.

62. B: *Inferial* is not a directional term used in anatomical positions; however, a similar term, *inferior*, means "below"; for example, thoracic vertebrae are inferior to cervical vertebrae. *Superficial*, *distal*, and *supine* are all terms that denote anatomical directions.

63. C: The CPT instructions specify that when a formerly established patient does not see a provider for longer than 3 years, they are considered a new patient upon return to the provider. A patient's transition from observation to inpatient care is not considered new; a patient seeing their regular physician who has moved practices is not considered new if it is within the 3-year time limit; and a nurse practitioner or physician assistant seeing a patient is considered within the same specialty and subspecialty as the physician, so the patient is not considered new.

64. D: In the CPT index, look for Blood Tests/Panels/General Health. According to the CPT guidelines, and in the instructions within this section's code descriptions, a blood panel must include ALL of the included individual metrics listed within that panel. Code 80050, for a general health panel, does include all of the listed required tests and is therefore the correct code choice. Codes 80047 are 80048 are for a basic metabolic panel only; 80053/85025/85004/84443 are for the individual tests performed within the general health panel, but they are not coded separately.

65. C: In the CPT index, find Dislocation/Elbow/Closed Treatment for code range 24600–24605. The correct code is 24605-51-LT to code for anesthesia as well as laterality, and modifier -51 shows multiple procedures. Next, in the index, under Fracture/Ulna/Olecranon/Closed Treatment, find code range 24670–24675. Olecranon denotes the proximal end of the ulna. The correct code is 24675, with manipulation, and, along with laterality modifier -LT, this code will be sequenced first according to the relative value unit order.

66. C: Look for Health Behavior/Assessment in the CPT index. Code 96156 is correct. Codes 96158 and 96159 are used for interventions, not assessments; 96160 is for assessment with administration of an instrument such as a health hazard appraisal.

67. C: In the ICD-10-CM alphabetic index, find Anorexia nervosa/binge-eating type/with purging. Code F50.02 is given and should be verified in the tabular list.

Weight loss code R63.4 is not used because weight loss is an integral element of anorexia nervosa; using a fifth-character placeholder of X is incorrect because a specific five-character diagnosis code is available. Code F50.2 for bulimia nervosa is not permitted in this case, as noted in the Excludes1 note in the tabular list.

68. D: In the ICD-10-CM guidelines, Figure I.C.15.a.1 is found in Section I, Conventions; Section C, Chapter-Specific Coding Guidelines; Chapter 15, Pregnancy; Section a, General Rules; Figure 1, Codes from Chapter 15 and Sequencing Priority. This figure is a flowchart describing how to properly code and sequence conditions within Chapter 15.

Other figures, flowcharts, and tables within the guidelines show coding and sequencing for conditions such as sepsis, poisoning, or those affecting pregnancy; properly using the guidelines' naming conventions will help coders locate the appropriate coding instructions for these and other conditions.

69. B: Although family and marriage counseling may potentially be a part of home health services, it is not a psychiatric service. Psychiatric services are offered by clinical psychologists, clinical social workers, and physicians specializing in psychiatry.

70. B: Status indicators MMM, 010, and 090 are all used to classify CPT surgery codes. Status indicator 000 is for endoscopies, not vasectomies or intrauterine device insertions. A complete list of status indicators can be found within the CPT surgery guidelines.

71. B: In the CPT index, look for Biopsy/Lymph Nodes/Open. Choose code 38510 for deep cervical nodes because the note specifies that the procedure was performed beneath the muscle. Code 38520 calls for excision of the scalene fat pad, which is not specified here; 38500 is for superficial excision, not deep; and 38555 involves additional neurovascular dissection.

72. C: In the CPT index, find Blood Banking/Frozen Blood Preparation. Of the code range given, 86932 is the procedure that includes both freezing and thawing. The correct reporting is 86932×2, for the two units needed for the surgery. Codes 86930 and 86931 are for freezing and thawing, respectively, but 86932 is a combination of these services and is the most concise choice. Code 86985 is for the procedure of splitting blood products.

73. C: The procedure performed was a mediastinotomy with a biopsy, represented by CPT code 39000. CPT code 39401 is reported for a mediastinoscopy, which is the insertion of a scope through an incision in the notch above the sternum. The ICD-10-CM code for a mass found on the chest wall is R22.-. Although the approach is cervical, the location of the mass is mediastinal, falling under the anatomical site of the trunk.

74. B: In the CPT index, look for Home Services/Activities of Daily Living. Code 99509 is the listed code and is the correct choice. Code 99507 is for catheter care, which is not specified in this case. Code 99600 is for unlisted home care and is not necessary since 99509 is the most specific option. For accurate procedural billing, and because more or less than the 10 recommended sessions may be needed, each session will be billed as it occurs; therefore, 99509 is billed individually rather than as a quantity of 10 sessions.

75. C: The surgeon performed a shunt system removal without replacement (code 62256), and modifier -78 shows that the same surgeon performed this unplanned procedure during the global postoperative period.

Code 62258 is incorrect because the system will not be replaced at this time.

Code 62252-78 is incorrect since the system is not being reprogrammed but removed.

Code 62256 shows the correct procedure code, but without its required modifier -78 for an unplanned return to the OR.

76. C: In the CPT index, look up Excision/Skin/Lesion, Benign. To report excision of a benign lesion on the face, code range 11440–11446 is used. Code 11422 is for the scalp, but the forehead is coded as part of the face. Modifier -22 is unnecessary since this is a simple procedure. Code 11312 specifies a shaving procedure, not an excision. Thus, for the excision of a 1.4 cm lesion, the correct code is 11442.

77. C: In the CPT index, find Anesthesia/Ligation/Fallopian Tube. Code 00851 is the only code choice. Further choices are shown by finding Anesthesia/Abdomen/Intraperitoneal. Code 00851 is the correct choice, with the modifier -P3 used to denote the patient's severe systemic disease. Code 00846 is for another sterilization procedure, a radical hysterectomy. Code 00921 is for a male sterilization procedure, a vasectomy.

Physical status modifier -P4 is for a severe systemic disease that is a constant threat to the patient's life, and this is not specified. Modifier -P2 is for mild systemic disease and thus would be incorrect to use for this patient.

78. A: Look in the CPT Index for the following:

Fracture
  Tibia
    Open treatment

The correct code choice for repair of the proximal end of the tibia is 27535. Laterality modifier -LT is added. Next, in the CPT Index look for the following:

Dislocation
  Knee
    Closed treatment

Code 27562, patellar dislocation requiring anesthesia, is a more specific choice than the codes for knee dislocation. Again, use laterality modifier -LT. In order of the highest relative value unit, the tibia fracture repair coding should be sequenced first. Modifier -51 is added to the second code to indicate multiple procedures.

Modifier -22 for increased procedural services is not needed. Code 27524 is for patellar fracture repair; the patient has a dislocated, but not fractured, patella. Code 27530 is for closed repair of a tibial fracture without manipulation, but this note specifies an open procedure for which manipulation was first attempted. Code 27552 is for knee dislocation, but since the procedural note specifies that the patella is the part of the knee that is dislocated, code 27562 should be used instead.

79. C: Code 31235 specifies a diagnostic endoscopy of the nasal passages and sinuses with sphenoidal puncture. A bilaterality modifier of -50 is not needed.

80. B: The CPT notes with the laparoscopy codes in the endocrine chapter (60650–60659) state that a surgical laparoscopy will always include a diagnostic laparoscopy, but that a diagnostic procedure can be reported separately using code 49320. This would be in special circumstances, but would not apply in a situation involving an allergy to anesthesia.

81. B: In the CPT index, look for X-ray/Clavicle. Code 73000 is the only choice given, and it will need modifier -26 because the radiologist is reporting a professional component within the ED facility. Code 73020 is for x-ray of the shoulder, but since code 73000 is of higher specificity for the clavicle, 73020 is not used.

82. A: Look in the CPT Index for the following:

Skin
  Tags
    Removal

Code 11200 is used once for removal of the first 15 skin tags, and add-on code 11201 is used once for the remaining 8 skin tags, for a total of 23 skin tags removed. Scissor technique, ligature strangulation, and several other methods of removal are all included within this code set, according to the CPT guidelines in this section. Modifier -51 is not needed because code 11201 is an add-on code and is therefore exempt from this modifier. Code 11305 is for shaving of lesions, a separate style of removal. Since the procedural note specifies scissoring and ligature strangulation, code 11305 would be incorrect.

83. A: The pericardium is the sac surrounding the heart. It consists of two layers: the outer fibrous pericardium and the inner serous pericardium. The serous pericardium consists of two layers, an outer layer called the visceral layer and an inner layer called the parietal layer. There is a fluid-filled space called the pericardial cavity between these two layers.

84. A: In the CPT index, find Thyroidectomy/Partial. Code 60210 specifies unilateral partial lobectomy, with or without isthmusectomy. Code 60212 also includes a contralateral partial lobectomy, 60220 is for a total lobectomy, and 60100 is for a biopsy procedure.

85. B: In the CPT index, look for Urinalysis/Routine. The correct choice for automated urinalysis without microscopy is 81003; confirm that all factors that the physician desires to test (e.g., glucose, pH, bilirubin) will be accounted for. There are several other code choices that are close but not accurate: 81000 is for nonautomated urinalysis with microscopy; 81001 is for automated urinalysis with microscopy; 81002 is for nonautomated urinalysis without microscopy; 81015 is for microscopic urinalysis only; and 81050 is for a urine volume measurement.

86. A: A radiologist may report either modifier -26 for the professional component or modifier -TC for the technical component, but not both. However, both a professional component and a technical component may be reported separately by different providers for elements of the same procedure.

87. C: In the CPT index, find Radiation Therapy/Treatment Management. The correct code is 77427, which is used once every five fractions over any time period. According to the CPT guidelines, when a series of radiation treatments has one or two sessions remaining after the initial fractions are billed, the remainder is not billed. Therefore, 77427 is the only code needed.

Code 77431 is only to be used if the full course of treatment is one or two fractions. Code 77469 is for an intraoperative radiation procedure, which is not specified here.

88. D: Stage 4 pressure ulcers may include necrosis of the soft tissue extending through all layers of the underlying muscle or tendon and into the bone.

89. B: In the CPT index, find Angiography/Cervicocerebral Arch. Code 36221 is shown and is the correct code since the catheterization of the aorta is nonselective. Code 36246 is for selective catheterization into a first-order artery, 36200 is for only the introduction of the catheter, and 36215 and add-on code 36218 are also for selective catheter placement.

90. B: In the CPT index, look for Anesthesia/Radiological Procedures. The procedure specified is diagnostic, making 01916 the correct code. The other code options are therapeutic. Codes 01922 and 01924 are for unspecified therapeutic procedures, and code 01925 does specify the carotid artery but is not diagnostic. In addition, the parenthetical note below code 01916 instructs that it is not to be reported with codes 01924–01926.

91. A: In CPT coding for E/M specialties, modifier -25 denotes a significant, separately identifiable service performed on the same day. The corresponding modifier for coding any other service is -59.

92. A: A hepatectomy is a surgical resection of the liver; the liver is one of the intraperitoneal organs within the upper abdomen. In the CPT index, find Anesthesia/Abdomen/Intraperitoneal. Code 00792 is the correct choice for partial hepatectomy excluding liver biopsy. Code 00790, for an unspecified procedure, is not the most specific option for the information given in the procedural note; and 00796 is for a liver transplant, which is not specified in the note.

For physical status modifiers, the CPT anesthesia guidelines provide instruction on how to select a modifier appropriate to the patient. The correct modifier for a patient who is not expected to survive without the operation is -P5. Modifiers -P3 and -P4 are for less serious levels of physical status, and P6 is used for a brain-dead patient who is an organ donor.

93. A: According to ICD-10-CM Guideline I.C.9.a., a cause-and-effect relationship between hypertension and CKD may be presumed. These two terms are linked by the term "with" in the ICD-10-CM alphabetic index. Unless a physician's documentation specifically states that the two are unrelated, they may be coded as related.

CKD and Lyme disease do not have this causal relationship, nor do disease of the mastoid process and heart disease, nor do diabetes and angina.

94. D: In the CPT index, look up Tattoo/Skin; codes 11920–11922 are referenced. For correct code selection, the total area is $10.75\text{ cm}^2 + 11.25\text{ cm}^2 = 22\text{ cm}^2$. Code 11921 is used for areas of 6.1 to 20 cm^2, and 11922 is for each additional 20 cm^2. Since 11922 is an add-on code, it is exempt from modifier -51.

95. A: In the CPT index, find Autopsy/Forensic Exam. Code 88040 is the correct code choice, and it does not need modifier 90 because the instructions state to use modifier -90 only for outside laboratory services. Codes 88000 and 88020 do not specify the forensic purpose; 88099 is for an unlisted necropsy procedure, and it is not to be used because a forensic exam is specified.

96. C: The desire for higher revenue is not a main focus of a compliance plan. Rather, accurate and faster payment of claims with fewer billing mistakes are likely benefits to using a compliance plan, along with diminished chances of a payer audit. Other benefits may include a decreased chance of violating self-referral and anti-kickback statutes, increased accuracy of provider documentation, and enhanced patient care.

97. D: In the CPT index, find Colonography/CT Scan. The options are codes 74261 and 74262 for diagnostic, or 74263 for screening. Code 74262 includes images processed before and after contrast material is introduced, making this the correct choice. Code 74261 is for CT scan without contrast material, which is included in the scope of 74262. Code 74280 is a colon scan using technology other than CT.

98. B: In the CPT index, look for Laparoscopy/Ovary/Oviduct. Under Occlusion of Oviducts, only code 58671 is referenced; bilaterality modifier -50 is not needed since both oviducts are included in the code. Code 58720 is for a surgical procedure, not laparoscopic; 58679 is for an unlisted procedure, but the procedure details in the note allow for more specific code selection.

99. D: In order to meet HIPAA requirements, the only individuals who may have access to protected health information are those whose jobs require it. Each doctor's office, hospital, or other entity must develop and implement policies to protect patients' health information in order to meet HIPAA regulations.

100. A: To locate an ICD-10-CM code, always start with the alphabetic index and then verify the code in the tabular list. Without verifying in the tabular list, correctly coding to the highest specificity of a potential seventh character is not possible. The table of drugs and chemicals and the table of neoplasms are very helpful tools in coding for poisoning, drug use, cancer, and other conditions; however, they are to be used in conjunction with the alphabetic index and tabular list and not as the sole means of locating a code.

CPC Practice Tests #3 and #4

To take these additional CPC practice tests, visit our bonus page:
mometrix.com/bonus948/cpc

How to Overcome Test Anxiety

Just the thought of taking a test is enough to make most people a little nervous. A test is an important event that can have a long-term impact on your future, so it's important to take it seriously and it's natural to feel anxious about performing well. But just because anxiety is normal, that doesn't mean that it's helpful in test taking, or that you should simply accept it as part of your life. Anxiety can have a variety of effects. These effects can be mild, like making you feel slightly nervous, or severe, like blocking your ability to focus or remember even a simple detail.

If you experience test anxiety—whether severe or mild—it's important to know how to beat it. To discover this, first you need to understand what causes test anxiety.

Causes of Test Anxiety

While we often think of anxiety as an uncontrollable emotional state, it can actually be caused by simple, practical things. One of the most common causes of test anxiety is that a person does not feel adequately prepared for their test. This feeling can be the result of many different issues such as poor study habits or lack of organization, but the most common culprit is time management. Starting to study too late, failing to organize your study time to cover all of the material, or being distracted while you study will mean that you're not well prepared for the test. This may lead to cramming the night before, which will cause you to be physically and mentally exhausted for the test. Poor time management also contributes to feelings of stress, fear, and hopelessness as you realize you are not well prepared but don't know what to do about it.

Other times, test anxiety is not related to your preparation for the test but comes from unresolved fear. This may be a past failure on a test, or poor performance on tests in general. It may come from comparing yourself to others who seem to be performing better or from the stress of living up to expectations. Anxiety may be driven by fears of the future—how failure on this test would affect your educational and career goals. These fears are often completely irrational, but they can still negatively impact your test performance.

Elements of Test Anxiety

As mentioned earlier, test anxiety is considered to be an emotional state, but it has physical and mental components as well. Sometimes you may not even realize that you are suffering from test anxiety until you notice the physical symptoms. These can include trembling hands, rapid heartbeat, sweating, nausea, and tense muscles. Extreme anxiety may lead to fainting or vomiting. Obviously, any of these symptoms can have a negative impact on testing. It is important to recognize them as soon as they begin to occur so that you can address the problem before it damages your performance.

The mental components of test anxiety include trouble focusing and inability to remember learned information. During a test, your mind is on high alert, which can help you recall information and stay focused for an extended period of time. However, anxiety interferes with your mind's natural processes, causing you to blank out, even on the questions you know well. The strain of testing during anxiety makes it difficult to stay focused, especially on a test that may take several hours. Extreme anxiety can take a huge mental toll, making it difficult not only to recall test information but even to understand the test questions or pull your thoughts together.

Effects of Test Anxiety

Test anxiety is like a disease—if left untreated, it will get progressively worse. Anxiety leads to poor performance, and this reinforces the feelings of fear and failure, which in turn lead to poor performances on subsequent tests. It can grow from a mild nervousness to a crippling condition. If allowed to progress, test anxiety can have a big impact on your schooling, and consequently on your future.

Test anxiety can spread to other parts of your life. Anxiety on tests can become anxiety in any stressful situation, and blanking on a test can turn into panicking in a job situation. But fortunately, you don't have to let anxiety rule your testing and determine your grades. There are a number of relatively simple steps you can take to move past anxiety and function normally on a test and in the rest of life.

Physical Steps for Beating Test Anxiety

While test anxiety is a serious problem, the good news is that it can be overcome. It doesn't have to control your ability to think and remember information. While it may take time, you can begin taking steps today to beat anxiety.

Just as your first hint that you may be struggling with anxiety comes from the physical symptoms, the first step to treating it is also physical. Rest is crucial for having a clear, strong mind. If you are tired, it is much easier to give in to anxiety. But if you establish good sleep habits, your body and mind will be ready to perform optimally, without the strain of exhaustion. Additionally, sleeping well helps you to retain information better, so you're more likely to recall the answers when you see the test questions.

Getting good sleep means more than going to bed on time. It's important to allow your brain time to relax. Take study breaks from time to time so it doesn't get overworked, and don't study right before bed. Take time to rest your mind before trying to rest your body, or you may find it difficult to fall asleep.

Along with sleep, other aspects of physical health are important in preparing for a test. Good nutrition is vital for good brain function. Sugary foods and drinks may give a burst of energy but this burst is followed by a crash, both physically and emotionally. Instead, fuel your body with protein and vitamin-rich foods.

Also, drink plenty of water. Dehydration can lead to headaches and exhaustion, especially if your brain is already under stress from the rigors of the test. Particularly if your test is a long one, drink water during the breaks. And if possible, take an energy-boosting snack to eat between sections.

Along with sleep and diet, a third important part of physical health is exercise. Maintaining a steady workout schedule is helpful, but even taking 5-minute study breaks to walk can help get your blood pumping faster and clear your head. Exercise also releases endorphins, which contribute to a positive feeling and can help combat test anxiety.

When you nurture your physical health, you are also contributing to your mental health. If your body is healthy, your mind is much more likely to be healthy as well. So take time to rest, nourish your body with healthy food and water, and get moving as much as possible. Taking these physical steps will make you stronger and more able to take the mental steps necessary to overcome test anxiety.

Mental Steps for Beating Test Anxiety

Working on the mental side of test anxiety can be more challenging, but as with the physical side, there are clear steps you can take to overcome it. As mentioned earlier, test anxiety often stems from lack of preparation, so the obvious solution is to prepare for the test. Effective studying may be the most important weapon you have for beating test anxiety, but you can and should employ several other mental tools to combat fear.

First, boost your confidence by reminding yourself of past success—tests or projects that you aced. If you're putting as much effort into preparing for this test as you did for those, there's no reason you should expect to fail here. Work hard to prepare; then trust your preparation.

Second, surround yourself with encouraging people. It can be helpful to find a study group, but be sure that the people you're around will encourage a positive attitude. If you spend time with others who are anxious or cynical, this will only contribute to your own anxiety. Look for others who are motivated to study hard from a desire to succeed, not from a fear of failure.

Third, reward yourself. A test is physically and mentally tiring, even without anxiety, and it can be helpful to have something to look forward to. Plan an activity following the test, regardless of the outcome, such as going to a movie or getting ice cream.

When you are taking the test, if you find yourself beginning to feel anxious, remind yourself that you know the material. Visualize successfully completing the test. Then take a few deep, relaxing breaths and return to it. Work through the questions carefully but with confidence, knowing that you are capable of succeeding.

Developing a healthy mental approach to test taking will also aid in other areas of life. Test anxiety affects more than just the actual test—it can be damaging to your mental health and even contribute to depression. It's important to beat test anxiety before it becomes a problem for more than testing.

Study Strategy

Being prepared for the test is necessary to combat anxiety, but what does being prepared look like? You may study for hours on end and still not feel prepared. What you need is a strategy for test prep. The next few pages outline our recommended steps to help you plan out and conquer the challenge of preparation.

Step 1: Scope Out the Test

Learn everything you can about the format (multiple choice, essay, etc.) and what will be on the test. Gather any study materials, course outlines, or sample exams that may be available. Not only will this help you to prepare, but knowing what to expect can help to alleviate test anxiety.

Step 2: Map Out the Material

Look through the textbook or study guide and make note of how many chapters or sections it has. Then divide these over the time you have. For example, if a book has 15 chapters and you have five days to study, you need to cover three chapters each day. Even better, if you have the time, leave an extra day at the end for overall review after you have gone through the material in depth.

If time is limited, you may need to prioritize the material. Look through it and make note of which sections you think you already have a good grasp on, and which need review. While you are studying, skim quickly through the familiar sections and take more time on the challenging parts.

Write out your plan so you don't get lost as you go. Having a written plan also helps you feel more in control of the study, so anxiety is less likely to arise from feeling overwhelmed at the amount to cover.

Step 3: Gather Your Tools

Decide what study method works best for you. Do you prefer to highlight in the book as you study and then go back over the highlighted portions? Or do you type out notes of the important information? Or is it helpful to make flashcards that you can carry with you? Assemble the pens, index cards, highlighters, post-it notes, and any other materials you may need so you won't be distracted by getting up to find things while you study.

If you're having a hard time retaining the information or organizing your notes, experiment with different methods. For example, try color-coding by subject with colored pens, highlighters, or post-it notes. If you learn better by hearing, try recording yourself reading your notes so you can listen while in the car, working out, or simply sitting at your desk. Ask a friend to quiz you from your flashcards, or try teaching someone the material to solidify it in your mind.

Step 4: Create Your Environment

It's important to avoid distractions while you study. This includes both the obvious distractions like visitors and the subtle distractions like an uncomfortable chair (or a too-comfortable couch that makes you want to fall asleep). Set up the best study environment possible: good lighting and a comfortable work area. If background music helps you focus, you may want to turn it on, but otherwise keep the room quiet. If you are using a computer to take notes, be sure you don't have any other windows open, especially applications like social media, games, or anything else that could distract you. Silence your phone and turn off notifications. Be sure to keep water close by so you stay hydrated while you study (but avoid unhealthy drinks and snacks).

Also, take into account the best time of day to study. Are you freshest first thing in the morning? Try to set aside some time then to work through the material. Is your mind clearer in the afternoon or evening? Schedule your study session then. Another method is to study at the same time of day that you will take the test, so that your brain gets used to working on the material at that time and will be ready to focus at test time.

Step 5: Study!

Once you have done all the study preparation, it's time to settle into the actual studying. Sit down, take a few moments to settle your mind so you can focus, and begin to follow your study plan. Don't give in to distractions or let yourself procrastinate. This is your time to prepare so you'll be ready to fearlessly approach the test. Make the most of the time and stay focused.

Of course, you don't want to burn out. If you study too long you may find that you're not retaining the information very well. Take regular study breaks. For example, taking five minutes out of every hour to walk briskly, breathing deeply and swinging your arms, can help your mind stay fresh.

As you get to the end of each chapter or section, it's a good idea to do a quick review. Remind yourself of what you learned and work on any difficult parts. When you feel that you've mastered the material, move on to the next part. At the end of your study session, briefly skim through your notes again.

But while review is helpful, cramming last minute is NOT. If at all possible, work ahead so that you won't need to fit all your study into the last day. Cramming overloads your brain with more information than it can process and retain, and your tired mind may struggle to recall even previously learned information when it is overwhelmed with last-minute study. Also, the urgent nature of cramming and the stress placed on your brain contribute to anxiety. You'll be more likely to go to the test feeling unprepared and having trouble thinking clearly.

So don't cram, and don't stay up late before the test, even just to review your notes at a leisurely pace. Your brain needs rest more than it needs to go over the information again. In fact, plan to finish your studies by noon or early afternoon the day before the test. Give your brain the rest of the day to relax or focus on other things, and get a good night's sleep. Then you will be fresh for the test and better able to recall what you've studied.

Step 6: Take a Practice Test

Many courses offer sample tests, either online or in the study materials. This is an excellent resource to check whether you have mastered the material, as well as to prepare for the test format and environment.

Check the test format ahead of time: the number of questions, the type (multiple choice, free response, etc.), and the time limit. Then create a plan for working through them. For example, if you have 30 minutes to take a 60-question test, your limit is 30 seconds per question. Spend less time on the questions you know well so that you can take more time on the difficult ones.

If you have time to take several practice tests, take the first one open book, with no time limit. Work through the questions at your own pace and make sure you fully understand them. Gradually work up to taking a test under test conditions: sit at a desk with all study materials put away and set a timer. Pace yourself to make sure you finish the test with time to spare and go back to check your answers if you have time.

After each test, check your answers. On the questions you missed, be sure you understand why you missed them. Did you misread the question (tests can use tricky wording)? Did you forget the information? Or was it something you hadn't learned? Go back and study any shaky areas that the practice tests reveal.

Taking these tests not only helps with your grade, but also aids in combating test anxiety. If you're already used to the test conditions, you're less likely to worry about it, and working through tests until you're scoring well gives you a confidence boost. Go through the practice tests until you feel comfortable, and then you can go into the test knowing that you're ready for it.

Test Tips

On test day, you should be confident, knowing that you've prepared well and are ready to answer the questions. But aside from preparation, there are several test day strategies you can employ to maximize your performance.

First, as stated before, get a good night's sleep the night before the test (and for several nights before that, if possible). Go into the test with a fresh, alert mind rather than staying up late to study.

Try not to change too much about your normal routine on the day of the test. It's important to eat a nutritious breakfast, but if you normally don't eat breakfast at all, consider eating just a protein bar. If you're a coffee drinker, go ahead and have your normal coffee. Just make sure you time it so that the caffeine doesn't wear off right in the middle of your test. Avoid sugary beverages, and drink enough water to stay hydrated but not so much that you need a restroom break 10 minutes into the test. If your test isn't first thing in the morning, consider going for a walk or doing a light workout before the test to get your blood flowing.

Allow yourself enough time to get ready, and leave for the test with plenty of time to spare so you won't have the anxiety of scrambling to arrive in time. Another reason to be early is to select a good seat. It's helpful to sit away from doors and windows, which can be distracting. Find a good seat, get out your supplies, and settle your mind before the test begins.

When the test begins, start by going over the instructions carefully, even if you already know what to expect. Make sure you avoid any careless mistakes by following the directions.

Then begin working through the questions, pacing yourself as you've practiced. If you're not sure on an answer, don't spend too much time on it, and don't let it shake your confidence. Either skip it and come back later, or eliminate as many wrong answers as possible and guess among the remaining ones. Don't dwell on these questions as you continue—put them out of your mind and focus on what lies ahead.

Be sure to read all of the answer choices, even if you're sure the first one is the right answer. Sometimes you'll find a better one if you keep reading. But don't second-guess yourself if you do immediately know the answer. Your gut instinct is usually right. Don't let test anxiety rob you of the information you know.

If you have time at the end of the test (and if the test format allows), go back and review your answers. Be cautious about changing any, since your first instinct tends to be correct, but make sure you didn't misread any of the questions or accidentally mark the wrong answer choice. Look over any you skipped and make an educated guess.

At the end, leave the test feeling confident. You've done your best, so don't waste time worrying about your performance or wishing you could change anything. Instead, celebrate the successful completion of this test. And finally, use this test to learn how to deal with anxiety even better next time.

Review Video: Test Anxiety
Visit mometrix.com/academy and enter code: 100340

Important Qualification

Not all anxiety is created equal. If your test anxiety is causing major issues in your life beyond the classroom or testing center, or if you are experiencing troubling physical symptoms related to your anxiety, it may be a sign of a serious physiological or psychological condition. If this sounds like your situation, we strongly encourage you to seek professional help.

Additional Bonus Material

Due to our efforts to try to keep this book to a manageable length, we've created a link that will give you access to all of your additional bonus material:

mometrix.com/bonus948/cpc

Made in United States
Troutdale, OR
12/01/2024

25570911R00113